Dedication

THIS BOOK WAS NINE YEARS IN THE MAKING. IT WAS MY PROJECT BUT there were many people who made it all possible. People, who supported, put up with and inspired me.

My daughters Shayla and Aislinn have been my greatest teachers in life. I am their dad but they have taught me more then I could ever impart to them. Thank you both for all the times you were there for and continue to be there for me. I am proud of you both and love you deeply. Your souls bring me joy and happiness.

Shelley is my wife who I met after this project began. I am blessed to have such a strong, talented, organized and supportive woman in my life. I am grateful every day for your presence in my life and how much you have inspired me to keep after this project, thank you. I don't know what I did to deserve your love but I'm keeping it!

Mom, it was because of your support and help I was able to make it to that first Ironman in 2004. You have silently taught me so many lessons throughout life and never ask anything in return. I have had the opportunity to be around a lot of strong and amazing people, none can match you in any way. Thank you for always supporting and encouraging me.

Dave and Tammy Noonan, two better friends a man could never have. I have been blessed by these two individuals in so many ways this small section could never hold all I would like to say. Thank you for always being there is not enough. I am proud to be your friend and always wish you the best in everything you do.

Dad, Grandpa and Grandma you have all passed but are alive in this book. Each of you had a part in some way shape or form in creating this project. My Irish heritage runs strongly through these Canadian veins and I am thankful that you all took so much time to help me become who I am.

And I would like to extend a special thank you to Kerry Wilson for her help editing the manuscript for this book. Your input and insight was much appreciated.

Table of Contents

Introduction

Upon a secret journey
I met a holy man
The Police, Secret Journey

I LOVE THE SAYING, "THE JOURNEY OF A THOUSAND MILES BEGINS WITH a single step." One needs to know or understand that they are on a journey. This is the story of my healing journey—only I didn't fully realize that I was on a journey. In the beginning, I believed it was a self-directed endeavour I was embarking on alone. By the end, I knew I had been called to make this journey.

My first step was actually a misstep. I gracefully (actually, it wasn't graceful—it was kind of ugly) fell off my bike during a Half Ironman Race, and that set a series of events into motion. I refer to that wipe out as the day God pushed me off my bike. You see, I was blind to Him, and He wanted to get my attention.

This incident resulted in a year long journey in which I trained for and competed in the 2004 Canadian Ironman Triathlon. I would discover that many lifelong lessons I had learned were a part of God's master plan. What I would be led into was an opportunity to develop a renewed mind and body. God was taking me where He knew I would follow, and on the journey He would heal me.

I was a broken man. I was unhealthy, and in many ways, lost. For many years I had suffered from depression. At times it had been almost debilitating, while at other times it was just lying under the surface, waiting to resurface. It affected my entire life, and it had an impact on the people I loved. For years I had longed to find a solution to this issue. I would find those answers on this journey.

A man's struggles can create his greatest victories. His lack of understanding can become his clearest insights. What confuses him can be the teachers that lead him to salvation. It requires a heart to find the value in what seems only to cause pain and suffering. What truly completes the journey is the teacher ... the wise one; the master. I was blessed that God became all of these to me. I had a movement of faith that started me on the path of this journey. Along the way I had to trust that what I was feeling and living was part of a greater plan. Then I had to listen and learn as I journeyed.

God wanted to be in a relationship with me. He opened my eyes, mind and heart to His incredible love. I need to make it clear that I am not an expert in the Bible or theology. I am just a regular dude who had an amazing opportunity to move into a relationship with God in a way that changed my life. God was the creator of this journey, and He allowed it to unfold and happen in a way that would grab my attention and take hold of my heart.

I sometimes think that when people hear the word "Christian" they think of perfection. Well, as a Christian I am far from being perfect. I actually don't strive for perfection, but I try to work towards excellence. I am a sinner who has many faults and things I struggle with as I move through life. I am telling this story because God has asked me to.

This is my story. I lay bare who I am and what I have done in my life. I am not the same man I was when I began the journey. I have been transformed in a way I never could have done on my own. God transformed my life when He entered into my space and time. He walked with me and still does. I am grateful to my Creator for the opportunity to tell how He healed me.

This journey began with a single step and ended in an Ironman race. I met myself along the way, and now my journey with God continues.

New adventures await, disappointments and lessons will be learned, and I will experience the joy and hope of a life lived with meaning. Above all, I will walk with a great mentor, coach, guide and friend in Jesus.

God Bless,

Daniel K. O'Neill.

Chapter 1

I'm Going on a Quest

"In the beginning was the Word,
and the Word was with God, and the Word was God."
(John 1:1)

I DON'T RUN, BIKE, SWIM OR EXERCISE BECAUSE I AM GREAT AT THESE activities. I do them because God made them great for the quest I would undertake—the quest that would return me to a relationship with Him. Just as God's Word shaped everything we know, His Word is shaping me. God has given me these activities to shape me. I didn't choose these activities or my life's course; I believe they chose me. God put me on a path. I have the ability to actively pursue my life as He defined it, or to allow life to act on me and keep me from the true path I was born to run.

The Word of God shaped me to be here right now in this space, writing these words. These are not my words; they come from God. God has allowed me to live each and every experience of my life for a specific purpose. It was God's will that I became what I am—that I run, swim, bike, exercise, and live as I have. Every time I exercise there is potential. Every time I exercise there is hope. I find opportunity in my training that I would not find in other pursuits. Training is about joy, pain, gain, loss, frustration, elation, and relationship with God. How the potential or opportunity manifests itself in my life is up to me. Every activity, breath, and movement is unlimited in its ability for me to grow in focus, discipline, and being alive. Each moment is an opportunity to create the world and myself all in one. I am an expression of energy, the same energy that created the universe. I am in relationship with God and His creation. If you tell me I am not, I won't care, for I have experienced the healing, loving presence of God in my life.

We have the potential to reach the highest expression of our true nature every moment we are alive—to truly live, breathe and flourish emotionally. We are also able to be in relationship with our Creator in His world of opportunity. God loves us deeply. Rather than feeling lost, depressed, and without hope, we can experience the life we were designed to have. It has become our human desire, brought on by societal conditioning and pressure, to just settle. Settle for the material comfort and pursuit of materialism. We buy into a marketing mindset of no pain or suffering, and bubble wrap ourselves in a cocoon while trying to eliminate what is bad, painful or dangerous. The energy spent on trying not to be rattled, afraid, weird, or different is immense, so much so that we actually forget to live our lives and enjoy our world. There are no guarantees that anything within the societal model or system in which we live will last. We spend more time pursuing security than living in relationship with the Spirit that gave us life. We serve ourselves and lose our connection to God.

Whether we know it or not, humans are on a quest. Do you live to maximize your potential? How about living to experience true, heartfelt joy? Do you get so much love out of life filling your heart that you just sit and smile for no reason? It is truly a quest to live your true nature and experience others who do the same. We all have our own personal quest, which is imprinted on our heart at birth. Your quest is as unique as you are. Just as there is no one genetically the same as you in this world, there is no one with the exact same quest as you. People are all hoping to achieve the same relationship with God in their quest, but they will never find it on the exact same path as you.

To be on a quest is to become infused with energy (as I write these words, I can barely sit still because I am so excited ... my energy is barely containable). This energy will fill us with discipline (the dirtiest word in the English language), focus, personal power, peace and joy (feel free to insert your own words here _____ _____). Your life will be altered when you pursue your quest and celebrate your true nature.

I personally don't want to leave any of my potential in the tank! Why save it up and not let it loose on the world? I don't want what "ifs" and "what could have beens" to haunt me in my later years. I want to be swinging in a hammock and looking up at the heavens through some trees, smiling and knowing I did what I was designed to do. I never want to settle for 'easy' just because it creates fewer problems in my lifetime. I have the power to direct myself on the path of my quest, and so do you. It's so easy to align your life with God through relationship with Him and to allow Him to work in your world. God knows what we require more than we do. God took the time to create and design each of us, and He designed us each with a specific purpose in mind. When we walk in relationship with God, our purpose is revealed to us.

When the energy of God's purpose for our lives is revealed to us, we experience life on a different level. Our inner world shifts and illuminates an incredible kaleidoscope of depth, knowledge, wisdom and love. We are able to create ourselves in an image so expansive compared to the societal image we are buying into. Our true nature is a wonderful way to live this life we are blessed with. This unconventional truth comes from living our quest through our spirit. Living this way aligns us with the Spirit of the God who created us. Have you ever been to the confluence of two rivers? At the point where they meet they are no longer separate, but they become one. We are never separate from God; we are the same spirit and body. The only thing that can separate us from God is how we live and think.

When we don't consciously choose to live our quest, we can become mired in the negativity of life. There is a negative societal quality to life that is magnified in the mighty media. This includes social media, which is just another venue for targeted bullying, attacks, non-privacy and so much more. This is a manipulative, financially driven way to exploit our human fear and desires. We need to be on guard against the forces that will keep us from trying to pursue our quest. It is a tough challenge to move through life in our society and follow our quest. More often than not, our quest will lead us down unconventional paths that will cause people to question us. Questing requires a huge resolve and desire to experience God in all aspects of our lives. The negativity contained in the daily media can take control of your energy and cause a great disruption in your life's quest.

Many people will see what we are doing as being selfish. It will appear our actions and intentions are selfish, because they may not align with societal conditioning and expectations. Our quest may conflict with what people deem is important in their lives, and this may scare them. The truth is, once you move into your quest and relationship with God you will become less selfish. Other people's perceptions should not shape you.

We can spend a lot of time and energy on what we want other people to think of us, even if it means going against our true nature in order to be liked, popular and accepted (remember high school?). We will choose paths that leave us feeling empty and lost as we just try to fit in. Our personal energy becomes blocked, and our frustration can cause many forms of illness and pain. We need to take back our energy and lives to live our true nature. When we live life as a quest and learn to use the higher power of God's energy available to us, we can be remarkable. I want to be remarkable, as defined by my own nature. It is a choice we can make every day. We must regain our will to live the remarkable lives we were given and are entitled to. A life lived in relationship with God is a life infused with the remarkable.

Our quest requires that we be disciplined in seeking the wisdom contained in the Word. It is a beautiful life when we live it with discipline (there is that dirty word again). The quality of our daily activities explodes with the opportunity to live a remarkable life. Being gifted with an awareness of God opens our minds and hearts. Oh man, what a wonderful world we have to live in and explore on our quest!

Life is contagious. It is short and offers us the chance to grow beyond our physical nature. The spirit which lies within is waiting to guide you on your quest. Join your own cause and become a disciple. God is calling out to you and wants to be in a relationship with you.

Experience what you were intended for. It really is a blast and will make you feel more alive.

Chapter 2

Life of Adventure

IS YOUR LIFE FILLED WITH ADVENTURE? DO YOU GET OUT AND HAVE FUN and go on unique journeys? Do you love to explore what lies within you and release it into the world? Or is your life filled with drudgery? Do you use narcotics and alcohol to escape the pain and misery of your days? Do you experience the same old tired, boring and non-motivational routine day after day after day? Maybe the question we should ask ourselves is, "What do I want my life to be like?" I think it is essential for us to take the time and dig around inside ourselves to find our true nature.

When I started to delve into the Bible, I realized how much adventure there is in God's Word. There is some crazy stuff that happens to people, countries and rulers. I am talking natural disasters, plagues, rivers that stop flowing, seas parting, the dead rising, the sick healed, and so much more. I have discovered that God wants us to live to our fullest capacity. We should not stymie ourselves because our parents, teachers, boss, or society feel we are suited to a certain way of being. Only God can show you how to live, because He designed you. I have felt and lived the power of my true nature, which God wrote on my heart at birth. I have also felt the disempowering energy of not living that nature.

If someone were to ask you in a job interview if you felt fully alive, what kind of inner reaction would you have? A job interview is an awesome place to express your true nature and sell yourself without personal limitations. I'm not talking about the outward face you would feel compelled to portray. I wonder how you would truly feel inside yourself at this question. Would the reaction feel good and come from your soul-felt truth, or would you just lie outwardly? I remember a time when I was part of the latter category. I would have been classified as part of the walking dead. Inside I was so miserable; I didn't feel alive. My life was a lie, and I hated the day to day things I was living. I made excuses for myself and blamed others for how I was living, because it was easier than taking personal responsibility. Life had become a boring chore; it was tedious and offered no excitement. It was a choice I was making without truly wanting to acknowledge that I was doing it. When I was aware that this was something I could control, I didn't know how to change the patterns and habits. It would take an adventure brought on by God that changed my world. At the time I began this adventure, I was not even aware I was on it! The end result of my adventure was an incredible transformation in my life. My world, and the way I viewed it, changed dramatically, and it all began with a call from God.

The year was 2003, and I had just separated from my wife of thirteen years. It was a happy time for me, even with the unfortunate side effects that go with an event like this in your life. It was a tough time financially, and it was even harder for our two daughters, which was extremely difficult for us as parents. I wasn't sad about the marriage dissolving, which says a lot about me and where I was at during that time of my life. On the contrary, I was feeling an immense amount of optimism and opportunity in my life. There was going to be struggle, frustration and some hard work ahead, but the mistake I had made by getting married was no longer going to keep me from being alive. It is sad to say, but true. I had been living an unhappy lie far too long.

This book was spawned by an incident that led me to the adventure that would change my life. Although the groundwork for the adventure had been laid throughout my life, God was now stepping into my time and space. I would be given so much creative liberty to pursue my true nature on this journey.

In July of 2003, I decided to travel to Penticton, British Columbia, Canada, where I would sign up for the 2004 Ironman Canada triathlon. It was a true leap of faith to be following this course of action. I was feeling compelled from within myself to go for it. I didn't understand it at the time; however, I was willing to just trust my instincts and go with my gut feeling.

With my daughters, Shayla and Aislinn, and the help of my mom, Betty, I headed to Penticton in August, 2003. From a financial standpoint this was a crazy idea. I was not in great shape financially, but this was one of those times I needed to be crazy.

For my entire life I had always done the safest thing. I followed the path of least resistance and the advice and desires of other people. My life and choices had been planned around what would be the safest course of action. Taking risks was not something I had been encouraged to do. I never wanted the discomfort of the unknown, or of what taking risks could entail. Taking this risk just felt right. Going to Penticton to sign up for Ironman Canada was one of the craziest things I could do in my life at that moment. It went against all of my reasoning and logic, yet it didn't feel unnatural at all. It felt right, and it felt good.

The trip was a nice little holiday for Shayla and Aislinn, who were dealing with the separation of their parents. I enjoyed being able to take them to a wonderful destination and treat them to some fun things. My mom came along to help me, and it was a nice way for all of us to spend time together.

Ironman Canada is a unique race in that you get to line up and register in person for the following year's race. As Ironman Canada 2003 was in its final hours, Shayla and I lined up at the Penticton Resort Hotel, where we would stay lined up overnight. On Monday morning at nine o'clock, registration for the 2004 Ironman Canada Triathlon would take place. Lining up overnight was fun and interesting. Having Shayla along to experience this ritual with me was awesome. We have some memorable experiences we can always laugh about and remember.

At eight o'clock Monday morning, Ironman volunteers walked down the huge line up and handed out registration forms. I filled out my form with great care and attention. Once it was completed, I just had to wait for the doors to the registration room to open. I was about to register to do an Ironman Triathlon. Wow! While standing and waiting to take the final step in the process, I was overcome by fear. The voice inside my head started to rear up with logic and reason.

"What are you doing here?" it asked me. "This is ridiculous; don't do this."

I was starting to listen and heard myself think, "Why am I here? I could just walk away right now and make another excuse."

This moment was fleeting and scary; it was a moment that felt as uncomfortable as any I had experienced in my life. The fear was paralyzing and horrible. It was a moment that reflected a lot of my life—fear based, afraid to follow my heart and not willing to risk taking any chances. But I was done with that. From deep within me came a calm, peaceful and powerful presence. A voice rose up and told me not to worry, that everything would work out. With the voice came an instant peace and awareness in that moment. All the fear washed away and left me. I stood next to Shayla, grateful for her presence, and feeling confident and sure. It was a feeling I wanted to hold onto and live like forever.

After going through the registration process and signing up for Ironman Canada 2004, I walked out into the warm, morning sun. I remember holding Shayla's hand and being full of hope. Man, I had not felt hope in my life for a long time. I felt confident that nothing was going to stop me from crossing the Ironman finish line the following year. I was sure in that moment that it would happen.

This wasn't about being cocky or arrogant; it was not coming from my ego. I was feeling a deep connection to the Spirit within me. I had been studying the Word and understanding how Christ had sacrificed on the cross for mankind, and that through his sacrifice I had inherited the Holy Spirit. In that moment, standing in the warm sun on a beautiful morning, I was filled with the Spirit. I was walking in the Spirit, buoyed by the energy of the Creator. Words cannot describe the feeling of knowing that no matter what happened over the next year, I would succeed in this goal. I couldn't fully see the plan, but God was bringing me to this mission. That was what I felt like I was on now—a mission!

I wondered about the inner pull I felt driving me to come and do this. The desire to be here had come from within me; it was not driven by my mind. A growing, inner compulsion to follow my heart was the catalyst for being a crazy man in this season of my life. Walking out into that sun and feeling the way I did didn't seem that crazy anymore. Nope, not at all. *Not* doing this would have been crazy.

It was an act of faith to listen to my heart and not my head. Here I was spending a lot of money that I really shouldn't spend (just signing up for an Ironman is big bucks), but that wasn't causing me any inner suffering. I was just feeling an amazing swell of energy in my heart that was guiding me. It was an adventure to come here and follow through with this idea. The experience had been so uplifting and clarifying. Now began the one year journey of my adventure to Ironman Canada 2004. The training, planning and hard work had just begun. But begun it had.

Chapter 3

UN!

Do not be conformed to this world,
but be transformed by the renewal of your mind,
that by testing you may discern what is the will of God,
what is good and acceptable and perfect.
(Romans 12:2)

I am not an expert in the Bible, which is important for you to know. Also, the purpose of this book is not for me to be preachy. When I use scriptures, it is because they make sense and having meaning to me. They have had an impact on me and my life, and are used as a guide in my relationship with God. Romans 12:2 will be a theme used throughout this book because of its relationship to my growth. I was immediately taken with these words and how they moved my heart. This scripture was a discovery that would alter my life. It was a challenge to my mindset and way of living. I love it when God challenges me to act and move.

My friend Kristine, who is a pastor (and a majorly cool one, too), helped me immensely with understanding the Word. Growing up Catholic, my exposure to scripture was limited to the "Priest dude" sharing the Word in his sermons. Kristine explained that the Word of God was alive. It was always possible to read a piece of scripture and find something new within it, as I often do. I would ask you not to think or feel that I am an expert in the Bible. I write this book because it's what happened to me. It's my experience of God entering my space and time. It's the story of how God healed me from my depression by leading me back into a relationship with Him. I am just relaying the experiences of a one year period that brought together many life time lessons imparted by God.

This chapter is going to require some mental stretching and calisthenics on your part. It's about a concept I derived on my own through Romans 12:2. This concept is a little off the 'beaten path.' Rather than follow the existing trail, I went bushwhacking. I didn't use a GPS or map; I just learned to follow my heart. Whoa, it's getting weird already! I promise that I won't use any mumbo jumbo or brain washing techniques here.

Conformity is an issue. I believe it creates automatons and eliminates humans. People stop thinking for themselves and acting of their own volition. I know this because I lived the majority of my life this way. On the outside I created an appearance of being unique, kind of rebellious and chic. Inside, I was a conformist—pure and simple. Growing up, I didn't create a mindset of my own; I was a follower for the longest time. I tried to elevate myself beyond conformity with my outward swagger, and I was semi successful in creating the image of a non-conformist. Mentally, however, I was a follower of others.

Looking back, I realize I didn't really think for myself. I followed the beliefs, attitudes and ways of my family and friends. Not that their ways or thinking were bad—I just never took the time to formulate my own mindset and way of thinking. I became a man who allowed others to form my opinions and ideas. I guess we all do that to some extent in our youth. As I got older, I found that I didn't follow my heart nor do what felt right for me. I followed what seemed to be the right course, because it was what people close to me were doing. This is not to say that I didn't benefit from some of this conformity, or that the thinking didn't help me. I have been successful and blessed in so many ways because of it all; however, deep down inside it never felt right for me. It was as though a big part of who I am was being subdued. My true nature was not the focal point of my mental processes.

On my adventure and journey to Ironman in 2004, I was shifting my perspective. I found there was a distinct separation between the mental habits I was following and my heart's constitution, and it was not working. Now I was experiencing an amazing transformation. This is what I can tell you: God was walking in my space and time, with me, in me, and through me. I even have to ask myself at times: What does that mean, man? When it was happening in the early stages of this adventure, I wondered what it meant. Could God actually have a physical impact or presence in my life? For me, the answer would be "yes," as revealed through the events and seasons of my life ahead.

God's impact would manifest in my life by how powerfully the Word would create a new mindset within me. God's Word moved me to a freestyle form of thinking, breaking down old patterns and habits. Through Romans 12:12, I was able to freely release my mental energy and create the mindset I desired.

UN is my mindset; it allows me to see the opportunities, actions and moments when God is present in my life. It came to fruition after I read a book by Paul Lemberg entitled *Be Unreasonable: The Unconventional Way to Extraordinary Business Results.*[1] This is an awesome book that made my mind spin in a positive and enjoyable way. I stumbled across the book one day while killing time in Chapters bookstore. This book caught my eye out of the hundreds of books on the shelves. Part of the book title was written in orange; since I am an orange freak, I didn't hesitate to read the inside covers.

There were five ideas on the first side of the cover, all written in orange: Be Uncompromising, Be Demanding, Be Critical, Be Outrageous, and Be Prepared. I didn't hesitate to buy the book. So what, right? Well, if you believe in random chance then yeah, so what. However, this was a time when my mindset was altering and changing. I took this as a moment designed by my Creator specifically for me. Remember, I was learning to understand the fact that God would walk with me in my space and time.

This was a book that would help me continue the mission God started with Ironman in 2004. In Romans 12:2, God teaches us that when we don't conform to this world, we will be transformed. God doesn't say that if we want to have our minds transformed we just need to spend a little time with Him. No, He says, "... *be transformed by the renewal of your mind, that by testing you may, discern what is the will of God ...*" We are transformed by God changing the way we think.

The scripture explains that once we have been tested, which allows God to transform our mind, we will see His pure and perfect will for us. We need to allow ourselves to give in to whatever God wants for us. There is a pretty funky point in all of this: God doesn't force us to do anything or to follow His will. We are free to choose; we can determine if we will follow or not. For a long time I didn't understand this truth, which had been right in front of me the whole time. God fully understood how much I required His time and presence in my own space and time. God was never separate from me; I chose to be separate from God. God created a new mindset for me. There had been plenty of acts of design in my life; God had been showing up in many ways over the course of my life. He was in books, experiences, people and places. God was showing me, leading me, teaching me and blessing me in quantum leaps. All around me were opportunities to grow daily in His wisdom.

I enjoy studying theory, philosophy and various self-improvement materials. Years ago, I decided that Romans 12:2 was going to be my focus. I was reading and studying the Bible and finding other scriptures that helped me. This one scripture in Romans was calling out to me. I felt an intense energy go through me when I would sit down and read it; I felt filled with power. It wasn't the kind of power that went to my head, however; this power went to my heart.

Romans 12:2 served as the stimulus for my UN concept. I realized that a refusal to conform to this world went deeper than just changing outward behaviour, which was what I had been focusing on up to that time. It is difficult to try and change conformist attitudes and habits by only focusing on the behaviour. I needed to have the ideal and wisdom of this scripture planted firmly in my mind.

God began to re-educate me, and I used UN as my guide. UNconventional starts with UN. The question, "why are things done this way?" is a great one to ask. In many places it is a red flag, as asking "why" may go against the status quo, or even threaten other people's security. I worked in a place like that for twenty two years. The same model and processes were in place for a long time. It was a conformists' resort where mediocrity was not only accepted, but was celebrated and rewarded. To make things worse, there was a heavy union presence in place. The UN at the beginning of union is a total misnomer and has no place in my UN concept. I have a lot of negative opinions and words to say about unions, but I will refrain. Suffice it to say, I don't like unions and wasted a lot of money that I had no choice but to give to them.

I worked with people who counted down the number of years, days and hours until they retired. Many of these people had contemptuous feelings for their employer and their jobs. Man, you are already dead, folks! That is not being alive in that moment. It was an energy sucking environment. I avoided many people I worked with because of their toxic attitudes and ways. I noted something funny during my time with that employer. The people who were the most vocal and outspoken about how much they hated their jobs were those who were the most opposed to change in the workplace! Rather than work and live to be remarkable, these people wallowed in apathy and accepted their fates. They actually made excuses about how they had no control and were being held down. Day in and day out it was the same script over and over for these people.

Life is so much more than just the societal surface we see. UN became my creative license to not be afraid. I started to think right up into the corners and along the borders of my box. I vibrated the area inside the box to create a new perspective and energy. I learned to walk with my eyes and mind open; it was my new art. I started to see that below the surface things are more calm and refreshing. The answer to a lot of our questions is not outside our box. We can diminish our own skills, talents and abilities by trying to look outside our own box. By all means do think outside the box. But if you take the time and listen to the energy inside your own box, you will find your true nature. God put it there to serve you on your journey and to fulfill your missions.

Here is my definition of UN: UN is a lifestyle, attitude and philosophy where conformity is to be avoided and eliminated. Through UN, I free my natural talents, gifts and skills that I received at birth from

God. As of October, 2010, the online Merriam–Webster Collegiate Dictionary describes UN as:

Prefix

1. Do the opposite of, reverse (a specific action)
2. a) deprive of: remove (a specific thing) from
   b) release from: free from

The same dictionary defines concept as:

1. something conceived in the mind: Thought NOTION
2. an abstract or generic idea generalized from particular instances.

I had not even looked up the definition of UN before I decided on UN as my philosophy. After reading the definition, it truly hit home how much this prefix fit with how I was trying to live. That is why UN works for me. I want to do the opposite of the past actions that were harming me. They came from a conformity mindset, and I wanted to be released and set free from these actions. The UN concept was conceived in my mind after I allowed God to work on and transform my mind. God removed my old thought patterns as I worked on listening to and following Him. UN is an abstract idea that creates more space in my mind to seek wisdom from God. UN was brought to the point of release within me on my journey to Ironman Canada in 2004.

I want to make it clear that I am not an anarchist or someone who believes in breaking laws. When I speak of being a non-conformist, I am not saying we should go out and start a revolution (unless you are being trodden on by a system that takes away your rights and liberties). My concept of non-conformity means not buying into the materialistic world we live in. Put God's Word and wisdom at the center of your life. Don't worship false idols and work only for your own gain. Live by God's law and plan for His creation. Serve what He intended, not what man has built for himself. I'm not saying we shouldn't make money, or enjoy the finer things in life. I like some materialistic things that bring comfort and adventure, but they should not be the focus and drive of our lives. Also, it is always good to have a charitable heart.

UN is a work in progress for me. I still find myself falling into old patterns and habits, which drives me mad, but I have a peace now that I know what the process is. I no longer see them as a burden or major issues as my conformist past self used to. There is good juju following me, and I am allowing the Master of Creation to pull me along in my UN.

I have an issue with the status quo and the fear of change. Again, it is not just about being rebellious for the sake of rebellion. If the status quo no longer works, or fails to be effective, then why follow it? Why not reinvent the status quo, making processes, life or work remarkable! You have probably heard this where you work or live: "That's the way we have always done it." If you were to ask why, however, you will often get an arcane answer, or told to just do your job. It is a deflating way to work when things never change or grow. Life is too short to settle for mediocrity and not even try to be remarkable.

The world is changing quicker than the old status quo can handle. Companies, people, organizations and other entities are facing rapid developments and changes daily. How often do we see companies and people left behind because they would not change? If the status quo can't cope with changes and daily functioning, then it has no value. Making change can be a difficult thing to do, but difficult does not mean impossible. Even if you make one small change a week you can begin to recreate your life or workplace. It takes energy and effort, but it is well worth it.

This chapter will never be completed, because I will never be completed. I live daily for the challenge of finding my UN and expressing it in my life. I find great excitement in knowing that God didn't create us to just exist. God created us to be remarkable, and we all have it within us.

Chapter 4

Quest for My Vision

I HAD NO CLUE WHAT A VISION QUEST WAS UNTIL 1985 WHEN I WENT to watch the movie *Vision Quest*, starring Matthew Modine (an UNderated actor). Modine plays high school wrestler Louden Swain, who is pursuing an UNconventional goal. People who are close to Louden think he is crazy for even thinking about this goal. His buddy, Kooch, tells him that he is on a vision quest.

It was a movie that had an impact on me at a young age. It spoke to my inner drive and determination, and I saw qualities in Louden that I liked. He was not conforming to what people around him thought he should do, or what societal pressure dictated. I would follow a similar course many years later in my own life.

A vision quest can be described as an intense time of spiritual communication during which a person can find deep insight into themselves and their world. It is usually a traditional Native American rite of passage in which the individual can spend up to four days and nights secluded in nature. This is a period of fasting, often leading to a dream vision, which can relate to that person's destiny or purpose.

I analyzed the movie and Louden's character intently. What I saw was a passion for his goal, and a commitment to what he wanted without being swayed or dissuaded. The character in this movie was not just pursuing a goal—he was pursuing life. Of course, I saw that Louden was not conforming, which was huge for me. As I analyzed the character, I started to look at people around me. I observed people close to me and people who weren't so close to me. It was an eye opening experience; it was hard not to be judgmental, which was not the objective of the study in any way.

I observed a lot of people with no passion for life itself. They were passionate about material objects and status, and they would pursue the most expensive house and cars, and try and get that promotion at work. After the glow wore off, the emotional crash would inevitably occur. Then they needed something more. Man, I see a lot of two car garages with so much junk in them that can only fit one car!

Then it was time to turn the observation inward, and I didn't really like what I saw there. I was doing a lot of this type of pursuing in my life. I wanted the objects and status, but I was not pursuing life. I was letting life slip right through my fingers. It was a sobering and eye opening experience for me. As I looked back at forty years of living and this lack of life pursuit, I had an AHA moment! I saw the difference between randomness and design. I could connect the dots of my hobbies, pursuits, loves, adventures and challenges, which outlined a quest for my vision.

I could see in my mind's eye what and how I wanted to be. I honestly just wanted to learn *to be*. I didn't want to be in pursuit of stuff or status. I just wanted to pursue Dan, and be Dan pursuing life. I had never learned how to just be. I was tired of chasing a tail that lead in the same circle.

That blueprint, or vision, of how to just be was up there in my mind. As I have journeyed with God, I have seen it come more clearly into view. As my relationship with God grows I learn to listen, watch for, and live His lessons. Through these all I am more and more aware of my vision and how to live it.

It's a fusion of my past and present pursuits that has produced the vision. All of these pursuits were not just random chance happenings and fancies. Each had a specific purpose in the design of my life by God: Dan's life—directed by God. It was at this point in time as I was returning to relationship with God that all the waters flowing through my life began to confluence together and create a more solid path.

Life's lessons and God's path for me began when I was young and started to play hockey. Hockey was the first real passion in my life. I know—that's weird, eh? A Canadian kid who loved hockey! Hockey taught me many life lessons that I still use today. I learned how to be a good teammate, which is something required often in my work life. I have worked with many people who have no concept of team, or even realize that they are part of a team. I have also seen the negative impact this mentality can have on an organization. I learned to respect my coaches and learn from them and their experiences. I was lucky and blessed in my time playing sports to have some great coaches.

Then there was the passion of football—not to mention the extreme joy of releasing pent up frustration and anger from my youth. Sports laid the foundation for my character far more than school did. If anything, school stripped me of my character and drive. It was sports that allowed me to pursue the path God had decided would be best for my life and His purpose.

This may seem like a total twist and deviation, but please follow along. I love cargo pockets. At work, my UNiform pants have cargo pockets that allow me to carry different tools and stuff I require, such as my personal notebook, a pocket knife, a card holder and other stuff. I love camping and wear fatigues for the same reason. Looking back over the first forty years of my life, I saw that God was helping me put personal tools in my own cargo pockets. My passions and loves were opportunities to grow as an individual. Each one provided me with a designed experience and a set of lessons that turned into tools for future use.

Stressing that these passions and pursuits were not just random may seem redundant; however, builders need to understand how each tool works. The tools required need to be appropriate for the job. A design needs to be provided for the tools to be used effectively. Remember that Rome was not built in a day!

Life, if it is random, has no meaning or purpose. We would just be wandering aimlessly with no reason to go on. If evolution is true, then would not a species be able to de-evolve as well? One of the laws of physics states that "for every action there is an equal and opposite reaction." Does that not mean that we could just reverse course and de-evolve? Just watch T.V. or YouTube, and I will no longer need to make this point. When I look at the human being, I see something incredible. With all of the intricate systems within the human being, and the unlimited potential, evolution is a put down. It is a personal injustice to the human being. What I see is an incredible design, crafted with so many possibilities and gifts. I derive great energy and passion from the fact that I am so unique amongst so many other incredible creations.

My vision of Daniel is derived from the numerous tools God helped me place in my cargo pockets. The design of this vision was written on my heart at conception and put into action at birth. Across the span of my life, God has revealed and continues to reveal these tools to me through different seasons of my life. God continues to create tools for me to pursue my true nature and grow.

One of the first tools He gave me was the Canada Fitness Test. One day in 1973, my teacher handed out a pamphlet outlining the Canada Fitness Test. It was a program designed to challenge students and motivate them to be fit. Political correctness has since wiped it out, because it could demean kids, but that's a topic for an entirely different book, because it really ticks me off!

There were a series of exercises and challenges designed to test your level of fitness. I remember running all the way home, so excited about this test. I wanted to show my parents, because I was burning with a passion for this thing. I lived over a mile from school, and my feet didn't touch the ground all the way home. Something about the challenge resonated within me, and I was hooked. A person could achieve four levels of awards, depending on how well they performed. There was the Bronze, Silver, Gold and the Award of Excellence. I made my mind up that first day that I was going to get the Award of Excellence.

I trained daily for each event in the test. I can't even remember all the events anymore, because it has been so long. From the time I received the pamphlet until testing day, the test consumed my mind, body and spirit. On the day of the test I was a vibrating mass of energy waiting to be released. Mom and Dad told me to walk to school to save energy and not to run. I used all my restraint not to run and get there like I wanted to.

At school we had to sit through a couple of classes before it was our turn to test. I remember how difficult it was to focus on the subjects. I just wanted to get to the challenge. One test I do recall was called the flexed arm hang. We were required to grab a horizontal overhead bar. Your arms then had to be flexed with your chin suspended above the bar. I don't remember how long we had to hold for. I remember being so focused during this exercise in the test that everything around me faded away. I was in the zone. My mind, body and spirit were intent on this one remarkable moment and just being in the moment.

I achieved my goal that day and received the Award of Excellence. I had focused on a goal and then went out and achieved it. I worked at it, focused on it, and was disciplined in my pursuit of it. It was a time of great awareness in my young self.

Why would I consider this a tool? I can remember how this challenge resonated inside of me, and how my heart swelled with excitement and energy. It was a defining moment that taught me about goal setting, showed me my potential, and helped form my physical possibilities. I learned a lot about what I was made of and what brought passion to my world.

As I stood in the line-up to register for Ironman in 2003, I felt this same energy, enthusiasm and hope when I heard the Holy Spirit rise up from my heart. In that instant, when I knew all would be well, it was the same feeling I had when I received the pamphlet for the Canada Fitness Test. I had followed my heart, and it would help me go on to many great things for me in my life.

Another experience God has turned into a tool in my life concerns sexual abuse. From the time I was six years old until I was thirteen, I was sexually abused by a priest who was also my uncle. It is important to understand that the purpose of this book is not to judge the church or my uncle. It was a season in my life and has significance on my journey.

The abuse remained a secret until I was in my early thirties. No one knew a thing about it, and it turned out I was not the only victim. My uncle was a sick man who hurt a lot of people. It was something that had a major impact on me as a youth, teen and young man. I cannot begin to describe the shame, anger, hatred, pain and so much more that consumed my thoughts, actions and life. I felt so alone for so long that life was a misery. I had thoughts of suicide, many thoughts of revenge, and so many thoughts that were not healthy.

The worst part of that entire experience was not being able to separate the church from God. I was angry at and hated God for what happened. I tried to run as far away from Him as possible. I didn't turn to drugs or alcohol; I found solace in sexual release. Women were only a conquest for me to release my pain through non-intimate sexual contact. I even kept company with prostitutes, because they didn't care if I was cold and detached. Sex was just a transaction. Women were a way to deal with my pain, frustration and loneliness. I wandered along in a valley like this for a long period of time. I didn't care about my life or what happened to me. I kept up an outer façade of normalcy and pretence, but none of it was true. I was not alive; I had no use for life or what I could contribute to it.

The depth of my uncle's actions eventually came to be known. There were many victims, and their stories all flooded out. My uncle was eventually incarcerated and held accountable for his actions. He was a sick man who suffered from pedophilia, and I will never condone anything he did. Part of me had pity for him, though. Eventually he was accepted into a program for sexual offenders called the Phoenix Program. This program had been very successful rehabilitating offenders and returning them to society in a functioning capacity.

While he was incarcerated, I began to feel an inner pull and desire to confront him. I didn't want to lash out at him, though. I felt compelled to visit him to give him my forgiveness! It was a feeling that grew within my heart and radiated out into the rest of my being. Part of me couldn't comprehend this idea, but in my heart it seemed right. I needed permission from the doctors in charge of the program to meet with my uncle. I actually had to do an interview over the phone with the head dude of the program. He was pretty honest about his concern that I would come in and give my uncle an earful, or want to hurt him.

I simply stated that I wanted to forgive my uncle. Eventually, I was allowed to make my visit.

When I met with my uncle it was not like in the movies with two phones on either side of some Plexiglas. We sat in a quiet lounge where we would not be disturbed. I was glad to see my uncle was doing well. He never once made any excuses for what he did. Part of this program was to own your sins and accept responsibility. While we talked I looked into his eyes—eyes that I had never wanted to look into again because of the power they had once held over me. I told him that I forgave him; I will never forget the look in his eyes upon hearing my words. This man had robbed me of a great deal of my life. Sitting four feet away from him, I could see a physical release in his body when I said three simple words, "I forgive you."

Forgiving my uncle triggered an emotionally charged release of negative, dark energy from my being. I walked out of the prison a changed man. My being was renewed by the act of forgiving my uncle. I didn't have to carry that crappy, negative, life draining energy any more. I was now free. I felt so alive. The sun on my face felt wonderful. The air flowing into my lungs recharged me. My eyes saw colors of the kaleidoscope that I had not seen for many years while walking in my haze. I felt myself walking into this world as it was for the first time. I was no longer walking aimlessly. I had been reborn.

I had to be brought to a place in my life where the act of forgiveness was possible. I cannot remember any other act in my life that was as freeing as this one. I had looked into the eyes of a man I once hated with all of my being and wanted to hurt, and had seen in those eyes the release from his burden after hearing my words. I am a man who has hurt others on my journey. I have lied and deceived, for I—like my uncle—am not perfect. I only hope that anyone who I hurt or slighted badly enough can one day forgive me for my acts.

Can what happened to me when I was young be considered a gift? I now see it that way and have learned that through God all is possible. I would never wish this type of suffering on anyone. I get incredibly mad when I read or hear about these types of abuses still happening in the world. Learning to forgive someone who had hurt me was a tough lesson; however, it has helped me to find the value in all the people I encounter. I may not like everyone I have to deal with in my life, but God has presented me with the tool that prevents these people from having any power over me. Only God truly has power over my life.

I don't believe for a moment that God intentionally had my uncle abuse me. I can't explain why something like this would happen to me, or anyone, but it did. What I can do is explain how God can take anything in our lives and help us to learn and grow from that experience. God has unlimited power to help you and I, and I can tell you that I would not have overcome what I went through without God's power.

Chapter 5

Heart Awakening

"Guard your heart above all else,
for it determines the course of your life."
(Proverbs 4:23, NLT)

I HAD A LIFE ALTERING EXPERIENCE IN ONE MOMENT OF TIME IN 2003 that brought this scripture alive in me. It was this one moment that gave me the impetus to sign up for Ironman Canada in 2004. It was not a happy or pretty moment for me, but it turned out to be transformative. I didn't know it at the time, but this moment would start me down the path to a renewed relationship with God.

It was kilometre eighty-seven of the ninety kilometre bike leg of the 2003 Great White North Half Ironman Triathlon. It was a rainy Sunday in July, and I was cycling well in my first half Ironman in thirteen years. It had been raining pretty much all morning throughout this race.

I was starting to think ahead and prepare for my transition from the bike to the run, which was less than three kilometres ahead. The rain was falling steadily, but not hard, as I rode. I had started the ride off freezing because of the cool air and amount of rain that had been falling, but at this point in time I was comfortably warm and feeling strong.

The road surface at this section of the race was filled with pot holes and some depressions. Race officials had used orange paint to mark these hazards for the racers. Due to the amount of water that had filled some of the depressions, however, the hazards were not visible, as the water was now above the paint markings. As I was riding along at close to twenty-nine kilometres an hour, my front wheel went into one of these depressions. The tire lost traction, and the moment of my heart awakening was upon me!

My bike slid out to the right of me, and I fell towards my left. I stretched out both arms to brace my fall. The impact of my hands hitting the pavement sent pain shooting up my right arm into my shoulder. I slid across the pavement on both palms, and slowly rolled onto my right side as I spun to my left. The roll carried me over onto my back, and I ended up in a seated position on the road. I was wearing a pair of triathlon shorts and a racing singlet. I had copious amounts of road rash on my right side and back. My left elbow was bleeding badly, as was my right knee. Both palms of my hands were cut, scraped and bleeding and had some gravel in them.

I quickly stood up and began to check my wounds. My right shoulder was sore, but functional. I was not seriously hurt, and a race official who was right behind me when I fell checked me out. The biggest concern was whether I had hit my head, or if I was too injured to continue. After talking with me for awhile, the official told me I could carry on if I desired.

I had set a goal for this half Ironman. I was going to break six hours, which would be a personal best. I had been well on my way to achieving that goal until I had my bike accident.

As I climbed back onto my bike to carry on towards that goal, I seemed lost. Physically I was hurting and felt beaten. It hurt to hold the handlebars, and blood was now staining the handlebar tape. Mentally I was a hurting unit for sure. I was mentally beaten, my focus was gone, and my desire to carry on was quickly dissipating. When I reached the transition area a few minutes later, I was done mentally. I got off my bike, which a volunteer took from me at the dismount line. I had every intention of walking to my transition spot, gathering up my gear, and heading home. I was quitting.

Quit? Yeah, that's right, I was going to quit. Who could blame me for quitting? I was bleeding, and my body was covered in road rash. It was the right thing to do. What was the point of carrying on? This was not my day, I thought, so I would quit and race another day.

As I walked to my transition area, I caught sight of my mom standing along the fence. Mom had a concerned look on her face due to my appearance. I walked to where she was standing and ensured her that I was alright, because I didn't want her to worry. I didn't tell her I was ready to quit. I turned and walked back towards my transition spot, still prepared to quit. That's when a deep, calm and peaceful voice said, "Pain is temporary, quitting lasts forever." It was a quote I had heard Lance Armstrong make, and the voice was that of the Holy Spirit. I remembered that inner voice from when I was a youth, and how it had comforted and guided me.

In an instant I saw what quitting would mean. It was a self fulfilling prophecy I lived over and over. How many times in my life had I quit something? I could find an excuse that would appease the inner pain of quitting. Quitting bothered me, but there was always justification for why I quit. It was a pattern played out over and over in so many aspects of my life. Something stirred in my chest, and I swelled up with energy. It was an energy so compelling that it filled me with a renewed resolve. Quitting was not an option this time, Daniel! If I quit, it would negate all of my training for the past six months. It would mean I was quitting on myself, and I could not excuse that. I went on and finished that half Ironman. It was not a personal best (I would accomplish that the following year), but it was a victory for me. I remember the race director placing the medal for the race around my neck. It was a sweet memento that would end up framed and holding a special place in my heart.

I now refer to that bike wipe out as the time God pushed me off my bike. At the time it happened I wasn't aware of the impact, value, magnitude and opening awareness this moment would have on me. It was the moment God stepped fully into my time and space. My relationship with God was going to become the focus of my world.

That night after the race while I lay in bed, I played back the events of the day. Instead of being demoralized, upset and frustrated about the bike crash, I saw it as a victory. For the first time in many years I had gone beyond personal limitations. I had somehow awakened, but what exactly had awakened? The voice I heard in the transition area was not new to me, but I had not heard it for many years. That had been my choice; I had walked away from the voice, but the voice had never walked away from me. Because I had been unable to separate the church from God, I didn't want to hear the voice anymore. I was angry for the suffering of my youth, and I felt that God had abandoned me. I had made a choice not to allow God in.

When one energy source is not willing to let another energy source in, it will be stopped. It's like building a dam where two rivers confluence to stem the flow of one river into the other. I chose to stop the energy God was willing to give me from entering my life. I had built a dam in my heart. There was no valve opened within me to the source of creation. The energy that created the universe would never stop entering me, but I would not enter into unity with creation, or with God. I was not allowing the divine energy of God to touch, fill, or live within me.

Lying in bed, I felt my heart open. The energy that swelled in my chest felt so good. The inner water of my stagnant river had been released to flow through me. God had moved aside the fortress walls I had built around my heart. My heart had been awakened.

I drifted off to sleep, feeling alive as if for the first time in my life. I felt a compelling stirring in my heart that I couldn't explain. The energy of my Creator now flowed into my heart and released me from my own prison. My world, Daniel O'Neill, was in a different shape than when I had woken up that morning, and it was only the beginning of the changes God was creating within and for me.

I woke up on the Monday morning and went for a walk. It was a part of the plan to flush the junk from the race the day before out of my muscles. It was a beautiful, sunny morning, and I was not sore like I thought I would be. My right knee was sore, and the six stitches in my left elbow were a nice memento of the bike crash. My spirits, however, were soaring. I walked without a purpose, and wasn't even aware of my destination. I just walked the bike paths around where I was living at that time in Sherwood Park. I felt compelled to walk, drawn by the inner energy of my swelling heart. I had been released from a self-imposed incarceration, and this was an awareness tipping point.

My good friend and coach, Dave, had twice completed the Ironman Canada Triathlon in Penticton. His stories and passion for the race had stirred my old dream of doing Ironman. Dave had helped me get into what was possibly the best shape of my life for the great White North Half Ironman. Dave loves the sport, and he was great to be around because of his passion. As I walked I thought, "What's to stop me from doing Ironman Canada next year?" I could go and do it. The thought resonated with the energy in my heart. It seemed as though this was not just a wishy-washy thought. It felt to me that it was by design that my heart had been awakened, and I found myself contemplating doing Ironman Canada as an opportunity to keep moving in the direction I was feeling. I could find plenty of logical and reasonable excuses and reasons why I shouldn't entertain this grandiose idea, but that was the mental Daniel; my heart was not concerned with all those logical thoughts.

I had a new aptitude for the feeling I was experiencing as a result of my crash. I could stand to live an adventure and follow the peaceful, joy-inspired longing in my heart. I had not followed my heart so many times throughout my life. All I had done was follow the ways of this world, and that philosophy had left me feeling dead! No more, not this time, no way!

I followed through with my inner, heartfelt pull. It was my defining decision, and it changed the course of my life. I would have, and still do have, a lot of work to do in my life. I am a work in progress, and sometimes a work in stasis. It is a work I enjoy now; my life is an art. Before this time it was something I loathed.

I would renew my relationship with God and enter into a new pursuit. God had shown me my true nature, and I was aware that this was the true purpose of my journey. Ironman was a tool for my cargo pockets. It would be an amazing journey filled with wonder, joy, fear and success. It was an amazing year I had ahead of me.

Chapter 6

Energy

It is interesting for me to observe energy. If you want to see how people act, try to observe their energy factors—their posture, voice, facial expressions and how they walk. It was an important process for me to understand about myself. I learned a great deal about how much impact these things had on my energy.

Quantum physics is an interesting subject to me. If you were to ask me about the physics and math aspects of it I would be lost. I was never strong at math; I just couldn't wrap my mind around it all. What I love about quantum physics is that these scientists are interested in the truth. There is a saying that goes something like this, "We are not humans on a spiritual journey; we are spirits on a human journey." This, to me, is a quantum physics saying. We manifest an energy that is physical, but it's the spirit within which is our true energy, our true nature.

I was once a negative mass of energy. I was my own worst enemy and not a fun mass to be around. There were even days I was tired of being around myself, and it's not easy to escape from yourself. The energy I learned to live from was negative, nihilistic and fear based. It was a weapon used to cover up my insecurity and anger from the childhood abuse. It would end up being this energy that would consume me, not help me. It is an uneasy awakening to realize how negative a force you have been. One can either continue to spiral further down into negative energy and attitudes, or choose to leave behind that which will never allow you to manifest your true nature. It is difficult to change, but not impossible.

How do I want to live? That's a good question to ask oneself. I think it should be a course in the school system. We are taught to function on so many levels, but not many of them are human. Our entire system is based on functioning in matters related to economics, work, conforming to the ways of this world and sustaining the system. We need to educate our youth to be self-aware. The energy we are brought up in is controlled and directed towards societal goals. If you don't feel aligned with that system, you can be cast as an outsider. You may dress, look and act differently from the norm, but that often leads to false judgements and ostracization. Your energy does not align with the norm, which is not normal!

I first became aware of energy when I took up Tai Chi. I was in my twenties and was not looking for this angle of the art. My desire to take tai Chi was to learn its gentle movements. I saw how peaceful yet powerful these movements were. I wanted their paradoxical value in my life. I quickly learned that there is more to this art than I was aware of. The sweet surprise of the power of energy would become a passion in my life. The level this discovery will have on my life at the time is not yet apparent. At this stage, I am just excited about what I am feeling, learning and enjoying.

Movement is the transfer of energy. The majority of our lives are spent in non-mindful, unaware movement. Often it is a sloppy transferring of an amazing gift. Mindless movement and action is a human illness. We have become accustomed to comfort. Our lives have so many technological advancements designed to make life easier. I don't want an easy life! Life to me should be energized and filled with challenges. Yes, some difficult challenge is good for the spirit. Some fun challenges are also good for the spirit. It is energy that is the substance from which everything is created.

Often I hear people talk about how tired they are. Life is hard work for them, even with all the tools designed to make life less stressful and hard. The daily grind of all the materialistic ways of the world can be tough. Life can be unfair, but it doesn't have to be a chore! Unfortunately, though, there are conditions and ailments that do have adverse effects on people and their energy.

The human mind is a tool for our use in life. Training the mind in energy is not something we do a lot in the Western world. We have a lot to learn from the Far East and their philosophies in training the mind. I have grown to understand that my mind is the tool that will have the greatest impact on my energy. Energy can come to us from many different angles and forms. The beauty of humanity is the differences we all manifest. What I draw energy from may not work for you, and vice versa. The important thing is to know what works for you. To be aware of what will bring you energy and what will drain you of energy is important. Enervation should be a subject taught in schools to help kids get a head start on this important part of our lives. Through the years since my first awakening to energy through Tai Chi, I have become acutely aware of what works for me. I have also learned to avoid the things that don't work for me. We all have energy vampires in our lives. I do what I can to avoid these individuals and other energy draining things at all costs.

Whereas the mind is the control mechanism for our energy, the heart is the engine. The heart is where the Spirit of God resides and where the same energy that created us flows with the Creator of it all. We have a resource that we can tap into that will rejuvenate us. My understanding and education in the art of energy was a continual process through the years and seasons of my life. After growing in energy through Tai Chi, I found even more power for my growth in the art of Kung Fu. How amazing this next level of education would be.

I had huge awakenings and learned about higher vibrations in the energy curve by studying Kung Fu. I learned breathing exercises that have become a staple in my life. Through these exercises, I find new, empowering ways to connect with the universal energy around me. I consider the universal energy to be the energy that is God who created everything within the universe. Powerful, intentional movement and non-action through peaceful meditation brought me to a new understanding of my ability to control my own energy, and therefore to control my ability to give into that energy, which is God working through me. Life is an art, an opportunity to express our true nature into the world we live in. Energy is the quality control mechanism of our artistic expression. Not taking the time to foster and understand energy is no longer an option for me.

I want to express my individual art in a manner that is tied into the creation we live in. There is no greater work of art than the human being. We are created in the image of God. That screams to me of unimaginable acts, thoughts and chances to make the most of my energy and, therefore, my life. If you want to think you were made in the image of a single cell organism, have at 'er! I use to like distractions from my every day, mundane existence. Things such as television and pornography were mindless ways to waste time. It was by my own choosing that I opted to spend my energy in this fashion. If I hadn't learned the tools that enabled me to design the means to focus my energy, I would have become a human black hole.

Kung Fu changed the focus of my artistic powers to enhance my ability to focus my mind. There are things we are capable of as human beings that we rarely explore. The conditioning of conformity to societal norms often means not exploring our own, unique human diversity. Society is continually becoming more accustomed to detachment from reality through the means of material escape. I can't fully fathom not using this incredible machine God created in our human form.

I consider movement of the human body to be a form of art. Being specific in movement through exercise builds endurance and power, and helps to focus the mind and body in unison with the spirit. Training in this way, I learned to harness the pure power of my energy, which I believe is an art. It is not only through exercise that the art of movement happens in my life. I have learned the gentle peace of simply being aware and cognizant of how my physical movements impact my environment and myself. I try to move in a manner that creates a quiet and peaceful air about me. I want my body to exemplify my art.

It feels good to live a life filled with energy. I am able to pursue my vision, filled with the knowledge I won't be too tired or worn out. I have found ways to continually tap the infinite source of energy we all have. By choice and not omission, I am able to access parts of my mental focus and discipline (there's that dirty word again) that I have come to love. Why not live filled with energy as opposed to the other option? I don't like the nihilistic, negative man I used to be. It served no functional purpose and was not an expression of the art I am capable of. To have gained the freedom from this self-imposed prison was a blessing.

If I were growing up in this day and age, I probably would be diagnosed as having ADHD. What's wrong with kids being hyperactive? Why do we put them on drugs to calm them down? Because the system can't handle them not conforming to its ways, that's why! They must be medicated in order for them to be assimilated. When energy is not allowed to flow freely, it will eventually cause harm. I held in huge amounts of anger over the injustice done to me as a boy. Sports allowed me to release a lot of that negative energy, but not nearly enough of it. Over time I became depressed. Man, that was a dark period in my life. I never want to be that way again.

I had to figure out that energy is a choice. I blamed my past and what others had done for all I felt and became. Ultimately, it was my choice to focus on and live from negative energy. I have found how much easier it is to live from the higher level of God's energy that creates positive energy. For so long I hurt myself, which in turn hurt those I loved. So much pain and inner, disjointed and dysfunctional energy was being cultivated. I wish words could describe how alone I felt for so long, and all because I didn't focus my energy or discipline my mind.

I wish words could describe the new feeling of joy in my life. The journey to Ironman in 2004 was a spark of liberation for me and set me free from an energy purgatory. All my previous aptitude about energy would transform in a one year period. All the tools God had provided for my cargo pockets were now a focused pin point in God's plan for me.

Have you ever had a gut feeling you just trust and know is right? How many times did you not follow that feeling because it just didn't fit the societal norm? For far too long I carried the regrets of too many gut feelings I never acted on. Instead, I would succumb to societal pressure and do what was right for others, going against what I was drawn to do.

My energy from July 2003 until August 28, 2004 was focused. I was awash in the highly disciplined act of concentrating the energy that

I would not allow to be displaced. I was in control of my energy and in alignment with my Creator, God. What God did for me over this time period is phenomenal. I had everything I required provided for me. God created many amazing opportunities that I could not have created myself. I did a great deal of my training in the Canadian Rocky Mountains in the town of Canmore, Alberta. When my 1987 GMC Sierra truck gave up the ghost, my friends Dave and Tammy came to my rescue with a 1999 Honda Civic. It was an incredible act of friendship that floored me. I never once doubted that I would complete the 2004 Ironman Canada. From the moment I signed up, God was creating the means for my success.

My friend and coach, Dave, told me before I went to Penticton in 2003 to sign up: "If you have any doubts about doing Ironman, once you see it and are there you will want to sign up." Until I was there to experience Ironman Canada as a spectator, I didn't understand this statement. When I was there to sign up the week leading up to the Sunday race, I could feel the energy. It's a palpable and living energy that you can feel. The momentum of this energy picks you up and carries you in its arms. Once the day of the race was upon me, that energy had consumed and hooked me. Having been around the running and triathlon community for eighteen years, I had never experienced anything like it. There really was a cult-like feel to Ironman Canada (a healthy cult). This is not a brain washing or narcotic induced loyalty. This is the cult of eliminating self-imposed limitations.

The Ironman experience would change how I viewed myself. I wouldn't settle for mediocrity any more. Not that I was going to ever win Ironman Canada, or that I was better than anyone either, but there was no way I would settle for anything less than focused and disciplined energy in my life. Mediocrity is a blasphemy against the energy God provided me with. I had chosen for too long to dampen the light of the Spirit within me. Unlimited, creative, and nurturing, I have found the pursuit of energy a true passion. My life is a journey, a way to live my true nature. I believe that nature was etched on my heart by a loving, caring and mentoring God. My own purpose in pursuing energy was part of His plan.

God was relating to me all these years. In the years when I wanted nothing to do with God, He had a lesson in every movement. Energy is a connection to the highest level of love we can have, the love of God.

No energy I have ever experienced will match the energy I find in relationship with God. To experience the peace and joy I now do never seemed possible before I was pushed off my bike. There is no chance or happenstance in my world. All of my experiences are by design of the Creator, and He lives each experience with me, right by my side. It's the ultimate experience of clear and joy-filled energy to know what you pursue is guided by the hand of God. It doesn't mean feeling superior or entitled. It comes with deep meaning and reverence. I have been blessed to pursue the physical limitations of my mind and body with the love, caring, coaching and nurturing of my spirit.

I am lucky to have the balance in life that exercise provides. In my industry, mediocrity and apathy are the accepted norm. There is a lot of negative energy, incivility, and downright immaturity that inundates me with negative energy. I have to work with a focused and disciplined mind to avoid ending up as a negative mass of human being. Some days I succeed, but other days ...? I am also blessed to be around some truly amazing and inspiring people who have found a way on their journey to express their energy with high meaning and gusto. I crave being around people who don't impose limitations on their lives. It's nice to associate with people that have a passion for life and push through societal conditioning to truly live.

Energy is a passion I pursue. I am not perfect and can falter, but I will never waver. I continue to grow in my space and time. When that space and time includes conscious focus and discipline in my journey with my Creator, I am never lacking energy. Pure, simple and oh so nurturing energy.

Chapter 7

Moving Mountains

I LOOKED UP AS I RODE AND SMILED AT THE ROW OF MOUNTAINS AHEAD to my right. I began this ride in Canmore, Alberta, with my halfway destination to the west at Lake Louise. I had already climbed the switch backs up to Mount Norquay and descended them again. Just west of Banff, I exited off Highway 1 onto Highway 1A. With less traffic on this highway, I loved this section of road. I rode past babbling streams and creeks, which were among my favourite attractions on this route. The odd deer could be seen at the side of the road. My pace quickened as I rode past the "Caution—Bear In Area" sign alongside the road (if he was in the area, I hoped my body was too skinny for his tastes). No matter how many times I am in those mountains, they always have the same effect on me. Mountains bring out a reverence in me for my Creator. My heart swells with energy and love when in the mountains. I have been so lucky to have had many wonderful experiences in them.

It takes consistent, focused and disciplined (AGAIN!) training to do an Ironman race. This type of training can consume a lot of time and leave you with less time for other important things. There is a trade off in life, and one has to find a balance. I was fortunate in 2003/04 to have the opportunity to train in Canmore. A friend who lived in Canmore was kind enough to let me stay with her when I was there. I made every effort to get to Canmore as often as I possibly could.

Riding and running around this small mountain town was ideal, due to the many great hills for bike training. The great running paths led me to many streams, creeks and rivers. Surrounded by nature, I would have a peaceful time to train and enjoy creation.

At the end of a long ride or run I would drive to Banff, which is a short distance from Canmore. The Banff Hot Springs were an incredible way to relax and recover from these long training sessions—nice, hot sulphur water in which to soak my soar, tired muscles, and all around me, as far as I could see, mountains to nourish my spirit. I was literally playing in God's playground. I would go for hikes to remote places and just feel my energy vibrate with the beauty that was all around me. It didn't matter how many times I ran the same trail or route; I never got tired of the injection of vital energy.

I had the opportunity to rock climb one evening. I had been on indoor climbing walls, but never out in nature. I couldn't believe how amazing that experience was. The climbs I did were not dramatic or difficult, but the amount of focus required was intense. I do not recall many times in my life where my mind had been that singularly focused. The scenery was beyond spectacular.

On my forty-first birthday, I hiked up a mountain called Ha Ling. It was a hike I had done before. The panoramic view from the top of that mountain of the valleys around Canmore is so cool. The Bow Valley spreads out below you and offers tremendous viewing. It was above thirty degrees Celsius that day. After the hike, I went to a spot along the river and waded into the translucent water to cool off. I didn't have a lot of material wealth in my life that year, but my heart was filled with richness.

When I wasn't training or on other adventures, I was reading or writing. I was either at the Coffee Mine or a smoothie bar in town that served great food. The world of my heart, the inner landscape of the Spirit within, was being nurtured. I was living from a place within that had long lay dormant for me. The outer world of society and its materialistic focus was lost on me. Who needs drugs and alcohol when you have the love of God and the Spirit within? I just had to walk out into His creation and merge my energy with His.

As I was reading the Bible at one point, I discovered this scripture:

He said to them, "because of your little faith. For truly I say to you, if you have faith like a grain of mustard seed, you will say to this mountain, 'Move from here to there,' and it will move, and nothing will be impossible for you." (Matthew 17:20)

I found this scripture unusually perplexing; I wasn't able to grasp any meaning from it. It was something that spoke to me, but I just wasn't able to understand it fully. The word "mountain" stood out, but I was looking at it from a literal point of view.

My training forays into the mountains had two purposes. One, of course, was to train and prepare for Ironman Canada, which felt great. There was more, though. A second reason for spending time in the mountains was spiritual in nature, but I couldn't figure out what I was supposed to learn, or what I felt God was trying to teach me. From the time I was pushed off my bike and signed up for Ironman, I knew there was a God-driven purpose for entering the race. I was making incremental gains in both my training and my spiritual growth. Sometimes an athlete will plateau in their physical training, and it can be frustrating. The same can be said for spiritual training, as well. I would often find myself frustrated with the patterns and habits I was fighting to change, and the issues within and about myself that continually had me falling back to ways I wanted to leave behind. I would get increasingly frustrated, which just triggered old response habits I disliked.

It was two steps forward and one step back in my spiritual training. For days and weeks I would make progress and learn. I would grow in and grasp the lessons from God and feel healthy and happy. Then for days and weeks at a time … nothing! GRRRR! Just nothing—and it was frustrating and trying. I wanted it all and I wanted it now! Give me the whole spectrum now. Why wait? I realized there was a flaw in my way of thinking and believing. I wanted too much too soon, and with a great deal of change required. I was getting ahead of myself.

I needed to let God work on me and create the change. If I was to stand aside, power down my mind and let the Spirit within me shine, I would have greater spiritual success. I wanted control, to be in control, and to have control—and I wanted it now. Wait, that's it! I want control, and that is opposed to faith! Could it be that simple? I wondered. I was trying to use the control of man when all I needed was to have the faith of a mustard seed grain. Me, me, me was my focus. I was going to do Ironman. I was going to do the training. I was going to reap the benefits of it all. I was going to make the changes and control those changes in my life.

I had to stop and look at the real reason I was doing this race. I wouldn't be doing it at all if not for the grace of God! If God had not stepped right into my space and time to push me off my bike, I would not be on this journey. I would not have contemplated this whole thing if not for God crossing my time line. Space and time. God and mountains. Life and opportunity.

Daniel, I realized, *you are the mountain.* All the times I have wanted to change and grow. All the habits and patterns in my life that held me back. That was what this scripture was brought to me by God to teach me. If I had faith, true faith in God, nothing was impossible.

Man, it is such a drag to struggle and try it all on your own. Here I was training for an awesome opportunity in the Ironman Canada race, getting to do a lot of that training in the Canmore, Banff area of the Rocky Mountains, and doing so many cool and amazing things along the way. Yet I was still getting frustrated, but I didn't know why. Why be frustrated? My eyes and mind had once again been opened. I was not going to get where I wanted in life doing it the old way. I was the metaphorical mountain in the scripture. I tried to beat the mountain into submission. I wanted to will it into being Daniel and make it so. When the results weren't there, I would fall back into my funk and depression.

I suffered many years from depression. I took antidepressants to help me with the imbalance of chemicals in my brain. I knew it was a natural imbalance in my body; however, to me it was a plain and simple weakness. I hated taking those pills and having to rely on them to be normal. Up and down I would go for the better part of my adult life, continually trying to control something I couldn't. My dose of antidepressants medication was the lowest possible dose. It balanced my moods and helped me function better in all areas of my life, but I wanted to control me and not have to rely on medication.

This struggle was a continuous one for me. I would stop taking my medication because I was determined that I was going to rule my life. It was my right to dominate my own mind and life. Then the crash would happen, bringing on the dark moods and attitude. Life felt impossible, because I was not able to control my chemical imbalance. It was not something I could control; it was a losing battle waged by a man who couldn't give up control.

The funny thing was that I liked being happy! The world is a place filled with so much possibility, joy and wonder. Seriously, taking one small pill a night was not and is not a weakness! It made me a better dad, friend, employee and person when I did take it. I liked medicated Daniel better—much better. So what was going on with me, man? Why would I avoid what made me happy and more functional. I really needed to look at it and ask myself the bigger questions. Why did I need to be in control? The answer, my friend, wasn't blowing in the wind. It was about me being human. I was full of pride. My desire to be in control stemmed from my concept of being masculine, aware, and in control of my life; however, I wasn't able to control what was causing my depression. It was a lethal combination, and I was stirring it deeper and deeper.

I was learning how truly unaware I was of myself and my true nature. Pride was blinding me to the solution that I already had at my disposal. I was feeling something about myself that wasn't true, but that I couldn't let go of. I felt a sense of shame about being depressed. I was ashamed of my actions and behaviours, yet the desire to keep my control was creating those actions and behaviour. It took a lot of faith to give up this type of controlling behaviour. I had struggled for years to be in control. When I was a boy, I couldn't control what was happening to me. When I turned thirteen, I put a stop to what my abuser could do to my body, but my mind was never able to regain the control I so desired.

God was offering me a solution that allowed me to override the ways in which my mind had dealt with the shame I felt from being abused and having depression. Shame is a debilitating emotion that rendered me powerless for so long. I was trying to use my will to make the changes in myself that shame had caused. There was only one will in the universe that was going to make a difference—the will of God. I was giving up control when I signed up for Ironman Canada 2004. The one year journey leading up to the actual race in 2004 was incredible, and it proved that God was there and would provide for me when I gave up control to Him.

Looking back, I can say in all honesty that had it not been for the support of my Creator, I would most likely never have done that Ironman. From training in Canmore, to the financial resources, to a vehicle that would end up being possibly the greatest gift I ever received—I owed everything to God. I was not capable of creating it all in that time. Only through the grace of God did I achieve what I set out to do.

Faith takes work. God will provide us with the means, energy and resources to follow our path, but we need to do the work. God will never force us to take a path or act in a certain way. We have the choice to follow His wisdom and Word, which will guide us always and provide for us always.

The Rocky Mountains helped me to train for Ironman Canada. They provided me with great hills and inspiration on my journey. The spiritual energy and experiences I had in them throughout 2004 created in me a stronger spiritual bond with God. I learned that faith is a key part of the process in moving mountains. I needed to look inward and not outward for the change I wanted to create. It required giving up control of some things in order for God to create in me the necessary vibrations of energy to become that which He had designed me to be.

Chapter 8

Discipline

WARNING- the contents of this chapter
may contain obscene language and thoughts
of an offensive nature ... get over it!

IN A WAY THIS CHAPTER WILL BE A PARADOX. CONSIDERING I GO TO great lengths to speak about not conforming to the ways of this world, it would appear that a chapter on discipline would contradict many of the points I try to make in this book. I have to admit that I took great pleasure in the writing of this chapter.

It seems that the word "discipline" is the dirtiest word in our society. Seriously, all one has to do is look through the news and read the majority of what is called news today—politicians lying, cheating and stealing; professional athletes lying, cheating and stealing; top executives and union officials lying, cheating and stealing. This list could go on for a long time.

In schools, children cannot be disciplined. Society tries to use reason and logic to deal with poor behaviour. This has its place and can be effective; however, it is not and should not be the last tool used. More commonly, though, it is the first option teachers, parents and employers have.

I have worked in the same industry for twenty-seven years. Within this industry, there is a term called "Failed to Report." It is pretty self-explanatory. People have what is called a "Report Time," which is the time you are supposed to start your shift. Failing to report means you are late, tardy, or not where you're supposed to be. In our industry, a service industry that is time sensitive, failing to report is not good.

A person who isn't familiar with my industry may ask, "Is this a common occurrence?" The answer is that this is way too common. For some people, it is not just common, but a regular occurrence. Many people who do this don't seem to feel it is so troublesome a habit or behaviour! Ummmmm ... so the impact you have on your team (loose use of the word "team" here) and your customers appears to be not as important as your own personal lack of discipline! What your behaviour says is that you are unreliable and even selfish. You don't feel that your employer is worth all of your focus, dedication and effort. You don't even care that your behaviour creates in you a mediocre character that is selfish and thoughtless about the trickle-down effect you create in your work environment. Sorry to say, but you need to either change or move on. So you see, lack of discipline is a way in this world, not just in my industry, but everywhere you look.

I define discipline as, "An internal system of focus, behaviour, and beliefs that dictate your habits and patterns." If you derive all of these beliefs, behaviours and focus from the societal norm, chances are you will lack discipline. Lack discipline and you are allowing yourself to be a slave to the ways of this world.

I have not always liked or agreed with my employers and their ways. I did work two years in private industry for a friend named Scott. He is a man of principle and works hard at his craft. I do not include him in the class of the first sentence of this paragraph. My employers pay my wages, which has allowed me to live the lifestyle I have. Contrary to what unions like to proliferate, it was not a union that got me this lifestyle. I will not lie; I am not a supporter of unions and feel they create an environment of mediocrity. My lifestyle is a direct factor of my employer and my character. I owe my employer the respect of a disciplined character, and that's the bottom line.

If there was something illegal, immoral or wrong going on at work, I would need to speak my peace. It would be UNdisciplined of me to not do or say something. It would only enhance and create more of the mediocre nature and energy that exists in my industry. I feel blessed to work where I do and earn a living the way I do. My benefits, our equipment and the workplace itself are amazing. I want to be a person who daily creates a better service and image for my employer. I take pride in wearing my uniform and representing our brand. At the same time, I am representing myself and my inner image of myself and what I believe in.

Here is another example of the lack of workplace discipline in my industry. I work in a uniformed position that is supervisory, and there are other employees whom I supervise that wear a uniform as well. All of us are visible to the public. Everyone who becomes an employee knows of the uniform code and that they will be required to adhere to that code; however, many people in the industry fail to wear the uniform properly. The uniform is comfortable; it's not ugly, and it saves people a lot of money that they would otherwise have to spend on work clothes. Even so, some people feel that they are exempt from the conditions of employment that were explained to them by their employer.

People wear different coats, footwear, sweaters, pants, and the list goes on. Why did they agree to take the job? To me, a uniform sets you apart and raises you up. It identifies you as a unique individual within a select group of people. That uniform is what marks you as a professional. But, oh no—their personal constitutions override the discipline and respect they agreed to! They are negligent of fulfilling a condition of their employment, one they agreed to follow in exchange for their employer's loyalty. I wonder in how many other areas of their lives they are cutting corners. When I put on my uniform, I take pride in my job, my employer and in representing my peers in the workplace.

Discipline is an opportunity to become the best person you can be. It is a choice between mediocrity and unparalleled art, and the art is you. As a society, the politically correct attitude of not infringing on people's rights has swayed the scales so far out of balance, it is becoming scary. I work in the transportation industry; my driver's license is my livelihood. Driving is a profession, not just a means to an end. Driving is a privilege and not a right. My license is a privilege that offers me many different advantages and opportunities, yet daily I see things done on the road that show the extent to which people can lack discipline, a sense of community and humanity, and the ability to tell the difference between right and wrong.

I could go on endlessly about the human stupidity I see daily on the roads. Speeding, texting, talking on cell phones, running traffic lights— these are just a few of the many dangerous and selfish acts I see. People just don't have the discipline or common courtesy to adhere to the laws of the road. Yes, folks, they are laws—not suggestions, but real laws! In my opinion, people think more about what is convenient than what is safe and legal. It is more convenient to leave late and speed. There is never any traffic at that intersection, so it is more convenient to just run that stop sign. I will just park in front of this store illegally in a fire lane, because it is more convenient for me. Yes, I am breaking the law, but other people do it, so I am justified. So what if I am putting others at risk? It is my right as an individual; too bad if you don't like it. It's my right to be undisciplined and a hazard.

My wife, Shelley, is a professional driver. She takes extreme pleasure in the discipline of her art, and it shows. Shelley wears the uniform as per the conditions her employer set out and she agreed to. There are some aspects of the uniform she doesn't really like or care for, but she understands that she agreed to this as part of her employment, so she adheres to that condition. Shelley's character defines the discipline she uses to work and do her job. Shelley doesn't get complaints, traffic violation infractions or create other undisciplined issues in her work day. There are a lot of these types of employees in the industry. Working with them makes my job a pleasure.

It is not just in her work life that Shelley displays this level of discipline. As a matter of fact, I don't know too many people who live as focused and disciplined a life as my wife does. I am blessed to have Shelley in my life; I and many others benefit from her commitment to discipline.

Discipline is a beautiful thing; it is an art. I have had the great fortune of hanging out with a lot of disciplined people. I have been associated with disciplined people in my work, in fitness and in training.

Being around disciplined people is energizing, educational and highly motivating. These people all inspire and challenge me to develop higher forms of discipline in myself.

One of my favourite Bible characters is John the Baptist. John the Baptist was a rock star in his time. People were coming to see this dude and be with him on a daily basis. He could have had a big head and let his ego take over, but he never let his mission in life be compromised by a lack of discipline.

John the Baptist had the mission to prepare the way for Jesus, and that is exactly what he did. John didn't allow anything to come between him and what God asked of him. No amount of sway from people or the society he lived in was going to make John change his ways. John the Baptist was a model of discipline we could all take lessons from.

At its core, discipline is the ultimate in self-respect. I like myself and want to be the best person I can be in all areas of my life. Relying on other people to be disciplined for me is a cop-out. Expecting other people to be disciplined, but not having the same level of discipline yourself is a common theme in today's society.

I often speak to people I supervise in my industry about some aspect of their behaviour that needs to change. You would be surprised at how many times I hear adults say, "Well, so- and-so does it!" Seriously, are we in grade school here? It reminds me of that saying, "If someone were to jump off a bridge, would you jump, too?" You give up your personal power when you are not disciplined. A lack of discipline is not in your best interests, and it will eventually have an impact on your health. Letting others be responsible for your life is a recipe for an unhappy you.

I know people who just find it easier to defer all areas of responsibility to other people. Then they will complain that they are stuck in dead-end jobs, unhealthy relationships, or that things in life never go how they hoped. Discipline is a way to focus and direct the abundant energy we each have. Discipline takes energy, and like a laser it creates a powerful force. When a person decides to harness their energy and be responsible, discipline becomes a quality control mechanism: if this works, I will continue to use this in my life; if this doesn't work, and has no value in my life, I am not going to practise it any more.

Discipline will be different for different people. As of January, 2011, the online Merriam-Webster Dictionary uses a number of words to define discipline: " instruction," "a field of study," "training," "control," "gained obedience" (oh man, that is another dirty word—obedience), "orderly or prescribed conduct," "a rule or system," and "order." There are more, but I think this is enough to get the point across.

Now is the time to define something about myself. I am not anarchistic, anti-system or opposed to rules. I just don't believe in blind obedience for the sake of conforming to a societal code that lacks morals, values and ethics. I am a big proponent of obedience and discipline.

People can be led to believe that giving up discipline is freedom. People can also be led to believe that following a certain discipline is the only way to behave and act. One only need look at religion, cults and unions to see these forms of mental control being leveraged. We all have a responsibility to the society we live in to be respectful, law abiding citizens. The pendulum of rights versus privileges has swung an awfully long way out of whack in our society. People become complacent and apathetic because of this ideology. It is an unhealthy pattern we have come to expect and are living.

Discipline, including the discipline that goes against the status quo, is the driving force of innovation. Organizations and systems want the status quo. They want people to conform to the system and not think or act in ways that go against the status quo. Disciplined people will invent the status quo. Those same people will write the status quo in the sand, not in cement. People who are disciplined do not allow personal limitations to become their truth. They are continually looking for ways to innovate and break through limitations.

The challenge to be disciplined is exciting. Allowing yourself to believe in your best self and pursuing that self is energizing. No one said it was easy to be disciplined; it often isn't. Often it is lonely, difficult, time consuming and extremely frustrating. The sad truth is it often takes less energy to fail than to succeed. Choosing to be mediocre is easier and takes less energy than being disciplined. In our society, it is safer to be undisciplined, because it is accepted as the norm and a human right. Sometimes there are greater rewards in society for being undisciplined. White collar crime is a prime example of people who occupy important positions being undisciplined and reaping great benefits from it. Ultimately, the truth of our Creator will override any and all other worldly ways.

We have a responsibility to the youth of the world to teach them how to be disciplined. Failing to give them corrective action for undisciplined behaviour does not do them any good. We have created a society where enablement is the standard operating procedure.

Discipline is not a negative thing or a dirty word. We all can become more disciplined in our walks, which is respectful to the human race and the planet we live on. People we encounter every day will become better when we live as disciplined individuals in their presence. It takes a lot of work on all levels of your life to be disciplined. We are human and we will make mistakes, but we owe it to God to live a disciplined life and to honour and praise Him. His love is the ultimate reward for our disciplined lives. Reflect what you truly are by allowing His light to shine through your life, lived in discipline.

I reflect on this in my journeying. I have chosen to believe in what Christ did on the cross, and to follow Him in my life. That makes me a disciple of Jesus. I have an example to follow of how to live a disciplined life. I am not expected to be perfect and exactly like Christ; however, I have a book filled with the Word of God to guide me in the ways of discipline.

Chapter 9

The P-TEAM and the Wise

"Walk with the wise and become wise,
associate with fools and get in trouble."
(Proverbs 13:20, NLT)

I'VE BEEN VERY LUCKY IN LIFE TO HAVE GREAT FRIENDS AND A LOT OF wise counsel. I like to think I have a few close friends and then many people I associate with. I think people have the perception that I may be aloof, arrogant and stuck up. Well, I'm not; I just let a select few into my heart. I take care of my personal energy and space, which may cause some of those perceptions.

I have been blessed with coaches and teachers who inspired me. They were strict at times and caring at others, and they were always there when I had needs. I learned many valuable lessons from these people, and I am thankful for their time and wisdom.

I have a core group of people who have made a big difference for me throughout my life, and I need to mention them here. I would never have attempted Ironman Canada in 2004 without the influence and presence of these people. The wisdom and drive in their lives influenced me to be a person capable of following through on such a goal.

I'll start with my daughters, Shayla and Aislinn. They have both taught me more than I could ever have taught them. Even at times when I was less than a good dad and adult role model, they have both stuck by me. I am so thankful for the gifts they have both been in my world, and how they have taught me. Shayla is my oldest daughter, and I believe she is a wise old soul. She has shown me often and with passion how to live Romans 12:2. Shayla walks her own walk, even when it is a struggle. I wish I were more like her in many ways. I have always been proud of her and what she has tried to accomplish.

Shayla is a wonderful singer and artistic individual. She doesn't have a lot of materialistic views, and she seeks to help others. She has a kind heart that has struggled to find its way in this world. Life at times has been difficult for her, because she doesn't follow the ways of this world, and that can be tough. I love Shayla and who she truly is with my entire being.

Aislinn is my youngest daughter and a hard working, dedicated young lady. Aislinn works hard and follows her heart in life. Aislinn sets strong goals and creates a mindset to achieve them. There is a persistence about her that is inspiring. Aislinn enjoys athletics and has done well playing basketball throughout her school years. The determination and work ethic she displays has made up for any lack of talent she may have. This is a person who knows what she wants, and she goes after it. I love Aislinn and who she truly is with all my heart.

I would not have achieved some of the goals I have in my life without these two daughters who sacrificed for and helped me. It is hard to train for an Ironman, work full time and be a dad. Often I was not there for them while I was training. Rarely did these amazing daughters complain, and they have always been there to support me.

Due to circumstances and logistics, Shayla and Aislinn were not able to come to Penticton for Ironman 2004. Both girls made bracelets out of wool for me that year. I wore those bracelets throughout my training and during the Ironman 2004 race. On August 28, 2004, while racing, I looked at those bracelets often and thought about and drew strength from my daughters. Thank you both for being such great kids and people. In 2008 I did Ironman Canada again and both girls were able to be there with me.

My mom, Betty, is the strongest person I know. By strong I mean dedicated, resourceful, sacrificing, intelligent, hardworking, organized, willing, confident ... man! This list could go on a long time! If Mom was ever hurting or down, I never really knew it; she is a strong individual. In so many areas I can't even compare to my mom, and I admire her for her skills. I am happy to have her guiding example to aim for in my journey. My mom made some really difficult decisions for her kids, at a time when it was difficult for a woman to do what she did. My mom made a stand at one time that saved her marriage and her family. She was a woman who was ahead of her time and lived so many things when she was young that women today think they created. It took a lot of courage for my mom to even think the way she did at a pivotal time for her, my dad and her kids. I never knew or understood the magnitude of her will and drive at the time she chose a certain path. I have only come to understand over time how strong and resilient my mom was and still is.

The wisdom of my mother is so deep and indescribable. Her wisdom is words mixed with actions and great discipline. I wonder at times how much wisdom she has to give, as it seems so endless. I would never have made it to Ironman Canada in 2004 without the help of my beautiful mother. No amount of thanks can express my gratitude and appreciation for your dedication and help throughout my life.

My dad passed away in 1994, at the age of sixty, from cancer. I learned many great lessons from him that I have tried to emulate in my life. Dad was Catholic, and my mom had no issues with us being raised in that faith. It was this exposure to Catholicism that opened the door of my heart to God. I saw my dad at his worst and at his best. He was an alcoholic for the first twelve years of my life, and then he joined Alcoholics Anonymous and was sober for the final twenty. I witnessed that man make courageous and difficult personal changes to save his family.

I will never forget the day he sat us kids down at the dining room table and explained to us that he had a problem. I was too young to fully grasp what was happening, but I saw my dad teach me an amazing thing. A man can admit he has a weakness. A man can admit that he has to get help from others for his problem. A man can ask forgiveness for the mistakes he has made and then let people choose how they will react. A man can change his life with the right amount of faith in God and hard work.

I have many wonderful memories of the man who helped bring me into the world. Dad was a first generation Canadian, and I learned a lot about my family heritage from him. My grandparents on my dad's side both came to Canada from Northern Ireland. We had a great relationship with my Pa's family, which has been a grounding force in my life. My only regret is that my daughters never got to know my dad. I have a picture of dad holding Shayla when she wasn't even two years old that I treasure. Aislinn was not born before dad passed away. Life isn't always fair, but I believe that my dad watches over all of us.

I have two siblings who are both older than me. My brother, Kelly, is the oldest of the three. He is four years older than me. Kelly is a firefighter and owns a drywall company. I have always admired Kelly's work ethic and his dedication to his family. He always knew what he wanted to do when he was growing up, and he went out and did it. He is incredibly hard working in all areas of his life, and I have learned much from his attitude and mindset.

My sister, Peggy, is the middle child, and she is three years older than me. Peggy and I have been very close throughout our lives, and I looked up to her so much while I was growing up. She was always there for me as a kid (and beyond). I could rely on her for so many things, and I am grateful to have her in my life. Peggy has an incredible personality. The song, "When Irish Eyes are Smiling," was written for Peggy. She has an enigmatic smile and way about her that just makes you feel good and want to smile, too. There was a time when she was the life of the party with all that crazy Irish blood in her.

There are two people I hung out with who helped to galvanize the mindset and attitude that got me to Ironman Canada in 2004. I was continually pushed by these two dudes; I love their attitudes, mindsets, work ethics and company. We would one day dub ourselves the P-TEAM (The P stands for PAIN!). The first P-TEAM member is my cousin, Derek. Derek is nine months older than me, and we were always close. He is the son of my Uncle Ned, who was my mom's oldest brother. Mom and Ned were close, so our families spent a lot of time together. Derek was the dude who swam against the current and never allowed any kind of limitations in his life to hamper his dreams or goals.

If Derek had it in his mind, it was as good as done. He just loved to have a challenge and do the work required to achieve it.

Being fortunate enough to hang around with an individual like Derek helps you learn a lot. There were so many things we explored because we wanted adventure and challenge. I ended up running and doing triathlons because Derek got into them and challenged me to try them. We were always challenging each other in some sporting event to push ourselves and see how far we could go. Derek and I were both competitive by nature, but between us it was a healthy competition. This competition between us fostered a deep connection that allowed us both to explore our deepest natures. I could not have accomplished the physical pursuits of my life without the wisdom I gained from Derek.

I met the second P-TEAM dude, Glenn, through Derek. Glenn is another guy who loved to explore his personal limitations through fitness and challenges. I spent copious hours training with Glenn and philosophizing about life at the same time. Glenn and I have had a close spiritual relationship over time that has grown along with our friendship. I trust Glenn in a way that words could never convey. Glenn is a true friend who has helped me in many ways that I just am so thankful for. I know that he was and will always be there for me. Glenn has provided me with inspiration and wisdom through so many wonderful experiences together.

There is wisdom to be gained through physical exertion. When you push yourself physically beside friends like Derek and Glenn, you get an attitude. It is an attitude of not wanting to let your friends down. You push yourself to be a person worthy of their dedication and support. While talking together during long runs or bike rides, you find lessons from training partners like these that will last a lifetime. I became a better man and person from the hours spent pursuing life with these dudes.

Dave and I are twins, even though I am six years older than him and we are not related. I met Dave in 2001, when he was Shayla's grade four homeroom teacher. Dave and I just clicked from the start. I worked nights at the time, so I would walk Shayla to school and spent a lot of time there volunteering. Aislinn was in kindergarten that year, so I was lucky to have the chance to be at the school a lot.

Dave and I started to run together, and he became another friend who would teach me many great lessons about wisdom. I would soon enlist Dave to coach me in my return to triathlon, because he had a lot of experience and knowledge regarding the sport and how to train properly. True friends like Dave are not just chance happenings in life. There was a higher design in place that brought us together.

One day in May of 2004, while driving to Canmore, my 1987 GMC Sierra truck blew its engine. The truck was not worth much, so replacing the engine was not worth it. I was struggling financially at this time, and things seemed very bleak for me. Dave and his wife, Tammy, had been trying to sell a 1999 Honda Civic for some time and had not been successful. They came to me with an offer that to this day still makes me so thankful for these amazing friends. They had me make a one dollar down payment, and I could pay them as much a month as I could afford.

Dave is a man of principle and has a sound spiritual foundation. Tammy is an amazing individual, who would often feed me and helped me with the girls where she could. Again, this friendship didn't happen by chance in my life. There was a higher power that helped me to meet these two friends that I am so proud to have in my life.

Dave helped me get to that first Ironman in 2004 with his wisdom and time as a coach. We have had some spectacular adventures together, and some great nights out as well (no drinking was involved on any of these occasions). Dave's spirit of motivation and drive has helped me grow as a person, and it keeps me feeling the inner fire of my own challenge-based mindset.

I haven't had too many people in my life who I considered mentors. There is one man, however, who has been an incredible friend and mentor. My buddy, Bill, is truly one of the kindest individuals I have ever known. He and his wife, Marg, have both been beyond kind and helpful to me in life. On two occasions during the time I was down and out and trying to change my life they let me live in their home. Bill and Marg are simple people, but they have a wealth of knowledge and capacity for life far beyond many worldly people I have encountered. I have been blessed to have these wonderful people in my life.

I have had some incredible conversations with Bill about life. It has always been a pleasure to sit and talk. I like to do a lot of listening when Bill is speaking. I find his wisdom for many things in life helps me to grow and see things from a unique perspective. I could never repay these two wonderful human beings for everything they have done for me.

So what's the point of a chapter like this? Another author talking about the important people in his life and what they mean to him? Yada, yada, whatever ... right? People do not just appear randomly in our lives. We are not just born to any family because of random chance, either. The theory of random selection has become a human cop-out. All these people I have written about are part of a specific design for my life.

People come and go from our lives in many different situations. Through his Word, God instructs us to walk with the wise. God is giving us a hint here that we need take note of. We will be exposed to many different people in our lives by design. God asks us to make choices through our interactions with all we encounter. How we choose to react, partake, behave and interact with them is up to us.

Each person I have written about has a specific reason to be in my life. I have had the opportunity to become enriched by their specific brand of wisdom. What I did with it all was, and still is, up to me. We have been designed to absorb massive amounts of information and process how to use that information. It is better to choose the Wisdom of God over the wisdom of this world (big "W" versus little "w"... Romans 12:2 refresher here).

None of these people are perfect, and I also learned some lessons from them on how not to behave. They are all in some way responsible for me getting to and competing in Ironman Canada in 2004. All of their combined wisdom has been helpful throughout my life so far. It has forged in me a mindset and attitude that helps me daily.

There were many other influential people in my life as well. To write about them all would take up too much space and become overbearing to you, the reader. I have walked with some fools in my life as well. Only by the grace of God did I avoid ending up on the wrong side of the law, or worse than that. It is good to have wise counsel in life and recognize it when you do.

Chapter 10

Breathe

I HAVE SPENT A GREAT DEAL OF TIME AS AN ADULT LEARNING HOW TO breathe. I discovered the power of intentional breathing in my training through the martial arts. We take our ability to breathe for granted. It is a physiological phenomenon we can use to create healthy, vital and powerful bodies. Before I started to focus on my breathing and train myself to do it properly, I was breathing too shallowly. I would not use the full capacity of my lungs, which in turn impacted many natural functions and held me back.

Breathing improperly and breathing dysfunctions can be contributing factors for disease. There is an unconscious as well as conscious aspect to breathing. The autonomic nervous system does many things during breathing that we are not conscious of; they are done unconsciously. Conscious control of breathing can bring many advantages to our daily life.

I mentioned earlier that I have used meditation in my life. The easiest form of meditation for me is consciously focusing on counting breaths. Inhaling is the first count of one, exhaling counts as two, inhaling three, and so on until I reach the count of ten. After counting to ten, I start over again. The objective is to do the counting without thoughts arising in the mind. Let's just say it is a lifelong practice and pursuit. An important part of meditation is to breathe fully. Meditation requires full belly breathing and using the diaphragm properly. Shallow breathing does not have the same impact and productivity in meditation.

Breathing comprises every aspect of our lives. When we sleep, our body remembers to breathe, although at a much lower rate. If our brain didn't control this function, we would die! Throughout most activities in our daily lives, we are not conscious of our breathing. Even when we exercise and eat we don't realize we are breathing. It is safe to say that for the majority of our lives we don't consciously focus on our breathing, and we may have habits that adversely affect our breathing that we don't know about or even understand. One of the biggest negative impacts on breathing is poor posture. I am not an expert in the areas related to these effects, so I am just going to put it this way: poor posture has a huge impact on proper breathing and can mess you up—BAD!

I learned through my martial arts training how to intentionally breathe throughout patterns. One has to focus on the intricate balance between the physical movements of the body and when to inhale or exhale. It takes precise thinking to achieve proper balance in the body to function at your highest capacity. This was true awakening for me; I had always just taken breathing for granted.

The by-product of the martial arts training was a greater awareness of my breathing. I started to take note of how I breathed in every situation—what would happen in certain situations and why it would happen. It was an interesting education in myself, and I was able to learn a lot. I believe one of the greatest discoveries I made about myself had an incredible impact on my health. I had been mentally taking note of my reactions in life and how they affected my breathing. I noted that when I was in stressful situations I couldn't control, or I thought were unjust, I held my breath. I would physically stop breathing or take the shallowest breaths possible.

Stress impacts each individual differently. I knew this about stress, but the effects stress was having on me didn't seem unnatural at first. I tried to just be aware of the impact stress had on my breathing and focused on trying to alter it if possible. I had some success, but for the most part I would more often than not revert to the old habit of holding my breath. I became bothered and annoyed by this habit, because I was making progress in my training and felt great about it. When I wasn't in the Temple training, however, I would falter. I like to get better at physical challenges, and I felt I wasn't translating the Kung Fu practice into my life. I would get frustrated, and frustration is a bad thing for me.

I needed to go deeper inside; I looked further below the surface to see what was happening. It required me to make a conscious effort to try and understand what it was that caused me to hold my breath in certain situations. I was becoming less than enthralled with this physiological process and what it was doing to me physically. It started to bug me when I found myself holding my breath.

I can't tell you what the exact trigger was for me. I found myself identifying situations that caused me to hold my breath and become really tense. My body would tense up and I would automatically hold my muscles in flexed readiness. My mental focus would narrow, and the world would disappear around me. I was in the fight or flight mode, with the object of my discomfort the center of my universe. These revelations led me to search the memory banks of my life. Why was I acting like this in these situations? What had caused me to freeze up like this and just stop breathing?

I found my answer in my young body being misused by a sick man. I need to make this totally clear. This book is not about me being sexually abused. It is not an attempt to gain notoriety, revenge or get back at people or organizations. It happened, and what I am relaying here was a by-product of it. This book is about how God healed me, pure and simple.

I remember how my body would respond when those acts of abuse happened to me. I would tense up as rigid as possible. I would take my gaze and pinpoint it on any place that allowed me to avoid eye contact. And I would hold my breath for as long as possible. That was my defence mechanism as a boy who could not defend himself physically. Okay, this makes sense now. In situations where I felt someone or something was unjust, my reactions were stronger and deeper. Sigh of relief—this was a good discovery. Now I at least understood why and could work on how to change it.

This kind of revelation was a relief. I could now focus on the root cause and change the effect. Having this new information made me feel better about my training and how I was doing. For a person suffering from depression, every little victory has a massive impact on the positive index. The immense power of breathing to change the physical impact stress had on me was so welcome. This was an important step in my own healing process. To fully have the ability to override the past and its control over my body and mind ... oh how good it felt.

I studied breathing in a non-scientific way. I chose to see it as a spiritual means to health and vitality, and I cannot stress enough the way proper breathing can improve your vitality. It was not just in the physical sense breathing impacted me. Mentally, the act of training and focusing on proper breathing was creating a man who was not lost.

I am going to the dictionary again, and the word is "foudroyant," which means to be stunning or dazzling in its effect. I thought long and hard about breathing and what it means to me in terms of my philosophy. I believe that breathing is more than just an act to live, or survive. It is an act that connects us to God, our Creator. Every breath we take is a powerful connection to the energy that created and sustains us, "... *He breathed the breath of life into the man's nostrils, and the man became a living person"* (Genesis 2:7b). Our very life, our very breath, comes from God's breath. I see the power and capacity of each breath I am lucky enough to take. That foudroyant breath ignited the human race. What am I capable of igniting with that breath in my lungs? I sure do want to find out. I see how so much of life is all intertwined, not separate and compartmentalized. Energy, true nature, heart, wisdom, breath and more yet to come! When I write sections of this book, I feel the excitement of my journey, and its impact swells my heart with energy. In those moments, I experience the deepest connection possible with God.

I don't want to waste my breath on mediocrity. The beautiful opportunity each day provides is too important to be mediocre. If I choose to be mediocre in my ways, what image of myself do I portray to the people I encounter in my life? If we don't do our best for ourselves, then what's the point? I am alive and healthy; that is truly special, and I am not going to waste that.

Continual experimenting with breathing and breathing exercises has helped me become a stronger athlete. One of my favourite training exercises is called Temple breathing. It consists of assuming certain stances, breathing in and out forcefully, and incorporating arm movements to focus the power of the breath. Doing these exercises can work up a great sweat and focus.

The physical exertion and tension created by these breathing exercises is intense. I can feel my muscles strain and work hard. My mind becomes a laser-focused beam. Feeling the machine that God created work in this manner is exhilarating. A person can generate a lot of physical power using these exercises and techniques.

My Sensei told me that if I did these breathing exercises regularly, I would start to notice changes in my body. He told me that they could change my physical appearance and the composition of my body. I was a sceptic at first; however, time and practice have proven him right.

My Sensei never spoke about Zen in a direct way, but all through my training there was a deep undercurrent of Zen involved. Kung Fu is an Eastern Art, and its origins have some Zen roots, so it goes without saying it was present in the philosophy. Let us then examine being present in the moment, breathing and Zen. I am not an expert in Zen, so that is important to note. I just understand the power of living in the now (I cannot help but think of Dana Carvey's character, Garth, in *Wayne's World* saying the line, "Live in the Now!"). That is the truth of Zen, and what proper breathing does for us.

Breath is energy moving within the body. That energy can impact every cell we have in our composition. Directed, focused breathing can change the very nature of those cells. We can create health, wellbeing and so many things in our bodies and minds with mindful breathing. Don't give away your power by believing you have no control over your health and wellbeing. In his book, *The Biology of Belief,* [2] Bruce H. Lipton describes how each cell in our bodies has a memory. I believe that by choosing to consciously breathe with intention and awareness, we can change anything about ourselves. I believe this because I believe God is that energy, and He will provide what we require to change. With intentional breathing, we are connecting to the immense power of God in each cell of our bodies.

Breathing was a lesson God used to help slow me down. It was a way for Him to prepare my mind and body for the moment when I could move into the relationship with Him that I needed. I would never have grasped the depth of His presence and abilities until I could fathom being in the now. I had what I now refer to as societal mind. How many things could I think about at one time? How many problems, issues, and disasters could I solve at the same time? How many plans could I make? I was being so mentally counterproductive, because I could not slow my racing mind. In Zen, they refer to this as monkey mind.

Multi-tasking is a big thing in our society, but it diffuses energy and can create mental havoc. It is the creating of necessity so we can pretend we are important and productive. It is an unnecessary evil that strangles our minds and stymies our lives. But man, does it make us look important! By learning to breathe with intention, I was able to slow and control my mind. I took back my personal power and was able to see myself through the haze. I didn't want to do anything, other than master Daniel. Focusing my mind's energy on other things didn't allow me to do that.

We give away so much energy and personal power in our daily lives, because it has become the norm to do so. We are the exception in creation, and need to start respecting ourselves as so. God created us to have dominion over the world He created. We don't even have dominion over ourselves as a species. Proper breathing is our way to maintain our own center and be in connection with God. When all around us is going berserk and is out of control, we can maintain our self control and ability to function rationally.

In my profession, I am trained in incident management. Often I can be the first person at the scene of collisions or other incidents that can create panic, fear and non-rational thinking. Believe me, I have had some co-workers who just couldn't even get proper information across in these situations. In such circumstances, I need to remain in control and think my way through in order to protect people and property.

Staying calm and level headed can be difficult. There is a direct connection between breathing properly and functioning properly in these situations. The brain needs a fresh, continuous flow of oxygen to function highly. The ability to breathe properly and act accordingly is essential. An aware, focused, and oxygenated brain can handle many stressful and difficult situations because it is prepared. I would like to see the principles of the martial arts taught as part of the physical education curriculum in our schools. Kids are able to comprehend this stuff quickly and assimilate it into their lives. Teaching kids to breathe properly and live in the moment would really help our society in the long run.

I used to love coming home after my evening shift and look in on my daughters, Shayla and Aislinn, as they were sleeping. When they were infants and youths, their breathing was deep, calm and peaceful. There is nothing more peaceful than a sleeping baby. We all could benefit from that type of peaceful, natural breathing.

Athletically learning to use the full capacity of my lungs was beyond awesome. It helped to increase my performance, and that is important when training for and competing in the Ironman. I was able to focus more on the act I was in the middle of without that monkey mind flying all over the place.

There is a plethora of material on the Internet about breathing. There are technical articles, theories, and much more to help educate and explore a powerful physiological connection with pure energy. There are also many books about breathing as well. There is power in your breath beyond what you may comprehend or understand. Take the time to give yourself the chance to explore the full capacity of your amazing body. It doesn't take money or a lot of time to physically alter your breathing; it does take work, though. My words can never capture what it can do for you.

This is my discovery about breathing and Zen. I meditate, breathe and exercise to calm my mind. In the still of my heart, God resides and is guiding me. I don't practise Zen to get to a point or space where there is nothing. I do it to get to the point and space where there is everything. That space in my heart where all of Creation and energy is waiting is God.

Chapter 11

Pace

ONE OF THE BIGGEST COMPLAINTS I HEAR FROM PEOPLE WHO OFTEN have no energy is how busy and hectic life is. Time is a big constraint for a lot of people. The pace of life is hard to handle at times, for sure. Well, here is my answer for that problem—SLOW DOWN! Seriously, folks, how many activities for your kids are enough? Say "no" to all the work related requests and ambitions. Buy a smaller house that doesn't take a week to clean. This is a societal ill we impose upon ourselves; it is not imposed on us, but is our choice.

Remember how technology was going to improve our lives and make them so much easier? I think we should revisit that whole concept. Even in the business world, I don't think technology has created less work or more time. I think the opposite has occurred—more stress, less time, and more job dissatisfaction. This is only a small portion of this list of technology ills in our lives.

I know people who wear how busy they are as a badge of honour. They compete to see how many activities they can get their kids into. I wonder who this is truly all about. Is this for their kids, or does it make them look like awesome parents in society's eyes? Often, they don't care or see how much damage and pressure this puts on the kids. I spent a great deal of my life following other people's pace. I tried to do it in jobs, a marriage, and in social circles. It was disempowering and unhealthy.

DANIEL K. O'NEILL

When I was in high school, I started working in a big chain grocery store. After I graduated, I went to work full time in this chain. During high school it was a great place to work. I made good money, had some great social experiences, and worked with great people. When I went to work full time after graduation, things changed a lot. I had to change stores and made some great new friends in the process. Productivity became a much higher priority at this bigger store, which had a manager with a bigger ego. This manager was a rock star in the industry, and he expected everyone in his store to be as well. When I work at things I am meticulous; I don't like to rush or be rushed. Well, I was not a rock star in this industry, and I was made aware of that often and unprofessionally. The pace had to be fast. I was not a horrible or a bad employee, but I just wasn't the prototype of what this dude and his cronies wanted.

"Bye, bye," I said. No money was worth being a target.

It was a great learning experience, but I didn't understand the lesson at the time it happened. I was immature, and it was easier to blame the people in power at that time. I would never have wanted to stay in that line of work, anyway, so it was not a great loss.

Many years later, in 2006, I was out on a training run on a nice summer day. I had learned by now that God would often show me opportunities, lessons or wisdom while I physically trained. God frequently used a simple, single word. That single word would lodge itself into my heart during my physical training, and it would become the focus of that activity.

On this one particular run, the word "pace" came into my heart and became a focus for me.

"Hmmm ...," I thought at first.

Pace! That is kind of obvious, isn't it? I mean, I am out for a run, and pace is important. The trick for me when God would enter my training space was to turn off my mind and just listen with my heart. The seed of a new challenge had been planted on that run, so my mission was to explore it. Why had God chosen to bring pace to my attention? What was I required to take away from this wisdom?

During any race of a physical nature, your pace is important. Every-one has a different pace, depending on genetics, ability and training. It is a skill developed over time, and can be learned the hard way sometimes. I recall many times in races getting caught up in the pace of others and blowing up. The start of a race can be a trap for this type of energy expenditure. The excitement and adrenaline kick in, and you can get lost in that energy and go out way too fast. Once that energy wears off, you can have a bad time the rest of the way, because you burned up a lot of energy too soon. As an athlete, I can achieve a lot and well know my limitations and pace. Pace may fluctuate from season to season, and can be affected by many factors. The biggest factor in my pace issues early in my training was stupidity.

As I thought about it, I started to see the purpose of this lesson by thinking in terms of my life. There were instances throughout my life when I tried to keep pace with the ideals and expectations of others. By now, one may see a pattern being established in my life. One where I don't follow what is best for me and my needs. I am not talking about being selfish and self centered here. What I am saying is that God created each of us a specific way. We all have a nature with which we are hard wired. I was so out of balance with my nature and what I needed to live and be who I truly was.

You can trace this thinking back to Romans 12:2 and not conforming to the ways of this world. Pace is a prime example of not getting caught up in the need to exceed the limit of your capabilities. Life is more enjoyable when we slow down and enjoy our time, not having to balance an unrealistic amount of pride.

I am so grateful for this wisdom imparted to me by God. I have become much more productive in all areas of my life by honouring my own, unique pace. One of the greatest aspects of my own pace was downsizing my material belongings. I had so much stuff, because it was deemed necessary. All it did was gather dust and take up space, creating clutter in my life. I still continue to work at this type of reduction in all areas of my life.

Life is enjoyable and filled with opportunities. I slowed down, which allowed me to focus on what was best for me. This pace allows me to be a better human in the areas of my life that matter most. I am a slow moving and thinking human being. I am fine with that, and I am happy to go slow. I am six foot three inches tall with long legs, so often when I walk with people they are much faster than I am. I don't like to rush at anything, really—especially walking. I can walk with purpose, but I don't have to walk fast. I just find that I am naturally slow, in a way that is not negative.

Finding my pace allowed me to weed out the things in life that just had no necessary place. I had so much stuff that I was being bogged down by it, and I didn't have time for the things that were important. That is not living; that is being a slave to things that are not worthwhile. I feel for people in today's society who are tired and so strung out by it all, when they don't need to be.

I found another side effect from slowing to my own pace was that I liked myself a whole lot more. By weeding out the non-essential things in my life, I got to know myself for the first time in a long time. I could see for the first time that which truly had meaning in my life. I had more and more time for those things that mattered. I understood now, as well, how much freeing myself from the societal pace allowed me to focus on my relationship with God. There was more time for me to focus on scripture, prayer and just listening to or looking for signs of God. Slowing my pace allowed me to find these things much more frequently. Life for me became enjoyable, because I was in control of me. I could use my pace to deflect the way the world was trying to bring me into its fold. I didn't want to be in that fold, not the way society was racing around with all its needs and desires. I was walking in slow motion, and I was not unhappy or missing anything.

Chapter 12

Obey and Covenant (more dirty words)

I HAVE TO ADMIT, THIS IS BECOMING A DIRTY BOOK. ALL THESE WORDS seem to stab our rights and individualism straight through the heart, even when they actually uphold and define our individualism by allowing our true nature to shine brightly. I have decided to combine two words in one chapter. I was originally going to have an individual chapter for each word, but I didn't want to scare you into putting the book down and running. That word "obey" is scary stuff and can freak people out.

There are a lot of scriptures about obeying God. It is interesting that an action designed to free us from our own sinful nature causes so much rebellion. We follow our own way and trip ourselves up so often due to that prideful way of acting. God is the truth; He created everything. Talk about the ultimate engineer and building project! When we obey God, it frees us to live a life of unlimited energy, filled with inner peace and joy. We are connected to the source that will inspire, motivate, guide, coach, mentor and love us unconditionally. God is not asking us to obey Him just for His own kicks and giggles.

When we choose to be obedient to God, we are truly set free. This freedom is different from how we have come to understand the societal freedom we pursue. I am blessed to live in Canada, which is a democracy filled with an abundance of riches and rights; however, within this society there is still a great amount of disease because of the ways of the world. Check back with Roman 12:2—we can become obedient to the ways of this world. When we choose to be obedient to materialism, distraction, greed, envy, anger, etc., we lose that true nature God instilled in us at birth.

We have within us everything needed to thrive and succeed in the world. I mentioned earlier that we have the greatest teacher, coach, friend and mentor, who will walk with us individually in our space and time. Yet we are continually educated and formed to look outside of ourselves to the societal experts. We are supposed to keep the norm, even when it may be the absolute worst thing and keep us from all God intended for us.

Obeying God is not always easy; it can be extremely difficult and even painful. In our human nature, we can feel trials and tribulations that cause pain and suffering. In our spiritual nature, we need to take solace in our obedience to God. He will never forsake us or make us walk the walk alone.

God made a covenant with each of us. He promised to give us the Holy Spirit if we believe in what Christ did on the cross and accept Him as our Saviour. A covenant is a binding agreement; Christ didn't have to make the sacrifice He did. He chose it. We have a choice between accepting Christ's sacrifice, or obeying the ways of this world.

For so long my life was an example of conforming to the ways of this world. I wanted to find happiness and escape from my inner pain by pursuing earthly desires and pursuits. None of these earthly ways ever satisfied what I truly longed for, or even came close to easing my pain.

I am a sinner. To deny that fact is to minimize the truth. It is a way to justify poor actions and decisions. I am human and therefore broken and not whole, and that makes me susceptible to sin. We have all been susceptible to sin since the garden and will be until judgement day.

I came to realize that we become what we obey. Those things in life we choose to pursue become our entire focus. What we focus on will become our master, and once that which becomes your master has a hold on you, it will not let go easily. I became obedient to anger and the desires of the flesh. It was so easy to use anger as a weapon because of the abuse. Man, it took an eternity to understand how that anger was not good for me! That anger consumed me and became the lens through which I saw everything in life. It was an ugly, false lens.

I still struggle with anger rising up in me during life's testing situations. It is so programmed into me that I just have it come up on auto pilot when I am frustrated. Frustration is the key for me. If I am frustrated, I need to realize it early, then there is hope it will not boil over. Each day I get better and better at creating alternative means to deal with life other than through anger; it is an exciting and awesome life to be living.

Ultimately, there is no excuse for me getting angry; it is a choice. I chose to walk a path with anger as my companion. Anger was a friend that allowed me to express all that was hiding within me. Unfortunately, people didn't know what the anger was about, so it was not understood. It wasn't a good friend, and it only made me angrier when people didn't understand. I obeyed what had come to control me for a long time in my life. I have to be aware and focused now not to allow this master to take control of me and my life. There are times I am not successful, and this has cost me. I can never take back the things I've done to the people I love. I will never be able to change people's perceptions of me due to certain actions. I have to live with that, and I make no excuses for what I did. I own it and only hope that anyone I truly hurt along the way can find it in their hearts to forgive me.

Weakness for the flesh has been a pursuit I obeyed in life. I was continually looking for solace in the female form, but not because I wanted to be intimate or in a relationship. I just wanted the sexual release they offered to me. I found plenty of women willing to oblige me, and I indulged myself whenever I could. If I couldn't find a willing partner, I would pay for a partner. I just wanted the escape and the release it allowed me for a short period of time. This pursuit gave me some escape time from having to live in my own mind. Like anger, though, sex began to control me. I was continually looking for my next opportunity to escape from my life. There were so many different options and stimulus in the environment to lure me. Sexuality and promiscuity is everywhere in our society.

Once again, I make no excuses for what I did. Everything was a choice, and I was not forced to be this way. Part of knowing you have problems is being accountable for your own actions and choices. For many, many years I did not accept any responsibility for my actions, and instead was at the mercy of the masters I obeyed. These things controlled me and dictated my life.

Obedience is misunderstood, in my estimation. It is one of those words that immediately makes us feel that we are giving up freedom, personal rights, and individualism. The moment you define something, it is hard to really see its truth. It becomes a societal way and is viewed as a definitive meaning. That is what the word "obey" has become—a definitively negative word to be avoided.

I think of the word "obey" as a sidekick to the word "discipline." To be disciplined is to become a disciple of a way, be it good or bad. Jesus' disciples obeyed him, and even they struggled with obedience to Him. To obey does not mean to be perfect. If we were all perfect, we would be living in the garden. I have learned to strive for excellence rather than try to attain perfection. I find on my journey with God that He only asks me to obey His wisdom. In relationship with God, we are not asked to be blind followers of a way and stop thinking for ourselves, which in truth is the way of this world, as we read about in the news every day (and in union newsletters; I have seen blind obedience in this type of organization that is truly scary). God just says, "Hey, Daniel, I know you. This is what I have laid out ahead of you so that you can experience life to its utmost as you were intended to do. Trust me, follow me by being obedient to this way, and I will give you more than you could ever imagine."

There is no command to do this and be this. God does ask that we have a good character and be willing to help others along the way. Being a good steward of the gifts God gave us is part of being obedient. We all have a different gift set from the Creator, and He will lead us to those gifts so that we may flourish. Whether it is a small gift in our opinion or a big one, in God's plan they are all beyond important.

Essentially, obedience comes down to how much you love yourself! Are you willing to give away your personal power to things that will not benefit you in the long run? Are you more interested in the ways of this world, which will steal from you your true identity? Obedience is a choice between the truth and that which is set up to limit you. Obedience will free you from things that will never benefit you. Have you heard the definition of insanity? Doing the same things over and over, but expecting different results! I think we have all been there and done that at some point during our lives. I know I followed the same patterns and habits for far too long in my life.

I want to be a person who experiences life and what it has to offer to the fullest. I have to sacrifice at times to allow opportunity to present itself, and other times I have to create the opportunity. Being obedient to a way is truly freeing, and it has brought me many opportunities I never could have created on my own.

Since I have learned to obey the voice of the Holy Spirit within me, I have become a happier and healthier man. I don't feel like it is an imposition to listen to the wisdom God has provided. Obedience is a way to create the life you truly want.

Chapter 13

Consider Your Ways/Intention

It can take a long time for an idea or concept to sink in. The tools God has been educating me in the longest are energy and intention, and I can be slow on the uptake.

Deciding to enter and train for an Ironman takes intention. I had to develop the determination to act in a certain way. In a nutshell, that is intention. As of November, 2009, it is also defined in the online Merriam–Webster Dictionary as: "the object for which a prayer, mass, or pious act is offered."

I was kind of an image guy before I did Ironman. I liked to talk about my feats and races. I never fully bought into wholly submerging myself into what it was to be able to do something like this. I was filled with pride and liked to be recognized for my accomplishments.

I floated through life doing just enough. I never fully applied myself to anything. It was a sobering time, looking at myself and the effort level in my life thus far. My report card was not stellar; there were lots of "room for improvement" comments on it!

God wasn't beating me up. When I was a kid, I thought that when I did something wrong a lightning bolt would strike me down. Since the time I signed up for Ironman, however, I have never once felt that God was a demanding creator. He has always just patiently waited for me to grasp what it is I was required to learn. The light of my ways was shining inwards for me to see. In order to fully understand the true nature God gave me, I needed to see how I was cheating on myself. I was talking a talk but not truly or fully walking it.

Haggai was an Old Testament prophet who was instrumental in the rebuilding of the temple in Jerusalem. The project to rebuild the temple began around 538 B.C. It was through the work of Haggai and Zechariah that the temple was completed in 520–516 B.C. People who had started the work on the temple eventually found other things in life to make their priority. They did not follow through on God's work. Well, God has a unique way of showing us where we may need to finish up or complete His work. Twice in the first seven verses of Haggai, God says, "*Consider your ways*" (Haggai 1:5, 7). God's house lay in ruins, while people of the time lived in nice, completed homes of their own. God reminded the people about the need to complete the temple, and that they should not be afraid for His Spirit was with them.

The book of Haggai is not a long book, but it has a powerful theme. When God asks us to do a work, He is with us. We need not be afraid of what we will face; God will prepare the way. The wisdom of this book applies as much to our lives today as it did when Haggai wrote it.

How we do this work is important. When I discovered my journey to Ironman was inspired by the will of God, I needed to get right in my head. God was working to transform me, so I needed to make sure my head space was available.

"Consider your ways" is more profound than those three simple words may relay. All of the wisdom, knowledge and lessons God was working to instil and provide me with were useless unless I made good on their value. God could not make me do anything if I didn't want to. It is not God's nature to force us; we always have the choice.

Upon reflection, I started to understand there are two types of choices in life. There are the choices we make without any thought or determination about the impact they will have. If I eat this bag of chips every day, then so what? Cheating on my spouse this once can't really hurt. Not performing my job with all my abilities won't hurt anyone. Making choices without thinking about their consequences or impact on health, finances, and other people is not considering your ways.

Then there are choices that we make with intention. I am going to sign up for Ironman Canada and do it. I will train properly, eat well, and live healthy to ensure I am fit. I will focus on this race for an entire year and create the energy and mindset required to achieve this goal. I will mentally, physically and spiritually put forth the time and intentional thought to do it. It takes less energy and effort in the long run to be intentional with our ways and actions. I began to discover through "consider your ways" that I hadn't done a lot of that type of thinking in my life.

I have more often than not been a reactionary unit. I would react to life as it was happening. I would allow the ways of the world to dictate my thoughts, feelings, emotions and how I was living. I tended not to think, but would rather be persuaded by society in the majority of my life's functions. This created terrible energy and a fragile emotional state for me. I played the victim for a long time in my life. I could justify it all because I had been abused. I was a victim! Life had been unfair to me, and it owed me for the horrible way I had to live because of what I had suffered through.

I was unintentionally making a choice by living this way. It allowed me to blame everything I did on the past. It was easy to create an illusory mental life that allowed me to give up my personal power. It created a crutch for me to lean on, and therefore not have to accept responsibility for my own ways. I can tell you how destructive and limiting this way of being is. The world had been far better to me than it had been bad. I had so many great people and opportunities in my life to be thankful for. I had a great family and friends who did many wonderful things for me. There was so much more to be grateful for in my life than what I chose to focus on.

It was only through intentional, focused and disciplined choice that I was going to make changes in myself and in my life. That first intentional choice was to have God as the coach and mentor in my life. Understanding how He could create the change I wanted, but was unable to attain, required faith. Part of this intentional choice to let God become the director and conductor of my life was giving up my perceived power. We all like to be the master of our lives; however, more often than not we are just pawns to society and its ways of controlling us for its purposes. God gives us true power through His desire to see us reach the potential of our true nature. I like to think of it this way: by allowing God to be the mastermind of my life, I was better able to gain mastery over myself.

The quality of my mind was changed by intentionally giving up control and allowing God to move me. My thoughts began to change; they gained a quality of hope and joy. I started to see the truth of God's creation around me, and realized how much more vibrant it was than that which society created. You may choose to call it positive thinking over negative thinking. In actuality, it was God creating my world for me. I became cleansed of an attitude that kept me from seeing the real world as created by God. It lives within all of us, just waiting to blossom and fill us with light. It is powerful, enlightening and nourishing in ways we can never create on our own.

It took deep reflection to consider my ways of spirit. I was kind of a fair weather Christian. I would put the effort in when I needed God; however, it was done more when I needed it than as an actual commitment and lifestyle. It was more about portraying an image than actually living it.

In the book of Haggai, the people were asked by God to complete the work of building the temple. As I studied the book, I wondered if God was asking me to complete the work on my temple!

> *Don't you realize that your body is the Temple of the Holy Spirit, who lives in you, and was given to you by God? You do not belong to yourself.* (1 Corinthians 6:19, NLT)

Your body is a temple! Daniel, have you been treating your body as a temple? Well, in certain ways maybe a little, but in many ways, no. Consider your ways! Oh man, does it ever end? So many angles and ways to consider that required my attention and action. I would like to say I was treating my body as a temple, but it was only a way to fool myself. I could do a lot better in all facets of my health and wellbeing. I was not honouring my Creator.

I admire and am in awe of the human body. There are so many intricate systems and other fascinating aspects of its design. The precision with which it operates is truly mind boggling. The majority of us just take our bodies and the amazing day to day functions they perform for granted. We don't nourish, rest, and honour them properly. The trinity of relationship with God is to submit our mind, body, and spirit to him. This body I have is on loan from the Creator, and He expects me to take care of it for Him. I have a responsibility to keep it healthy and productive.

I had a lot of intentional work to perform with my physical body. I was not eating properly the majority of the time. I wasn't hydrating properly, and my rest was not adequate. Yes, I was training myself physically, which was good, but the bigger picture needed tending to.

In April of 2004, I walked into a quaint little bookstore in Canmore. I love reading, and bookstores are special places for me. I wasn't looking for anything in particular. I just felt compelled to go in and look. Behind the counter in the new releases section was a book by Dr. Wayne Dyer called, *The Power of Intention*.[3] Coincidence? Well, I bought it. It is a great book on this subject. I highly recommend it to anyone looking for some insight into intention.

It can be difficult work to consider your ways. I have had, and know there will be, moments of frustration for me. I would have times of growth and success, but then would slip. It was a continual process of taking the time to think intentionally about my actions. It was only through intention that I would be able to overcome habits and patterns that were having a negative impact on my temple.

I intend to pack as much living and adventure into my life as possible. Life is short; however, it is an audition for a better life. I want to be alive for as long as possible, so that I can live with intention and serve my Creator. Truly take a look at this amazing creation which is the human being. Celebrate your temple every day by living through the act of design. You are not just some random chance happening.

Chapter 14

Why Would You Do That?

MORE THAN ONCE DURING MY TRAINING FOR IRONMAN I WOULD BE asked, "Why would you do that?" My standard answer would be, "Because I can!" I started to think about this response and realized how much it minimized what I was trying to accomplish. To complete an Ironman, you have to cover 140.6 miles in three different sports in less than seventeen hours. You swim 2.4 miles, cycle 112 miles, and then run 26.2 miles. It runs one event consecutively after the other, rain or shine, waves or still water, hills and flats. It is an endurance event that takes commitment, determination and a lot of spirit. One doesn't just wing it when it comes to Ironman. If you aren't prepared, you will pay a price. You need to be physically prepared for the rigors of this challenging course in Penticton. There is a lot of work that goes into training to complete Ironman Canada.

I wondered what my physical limitations might be when I signed up for Ironman. I had run marathons before and completed Half Ironman races; however, this would be a whole different beast altogether. It wasn't that I had doubt— it was more a fear of the unknown. Would I be able to put it all together and do this?

It requires commitment to train for Ironman, and I had added responsibilities. I was working full time, raising my daughters, starting fresh in my life after separating from my wife, and heading for divorce. Many times it felt overwhelming to try juggling all the stuff happening in my life. There is only so much time in a day, and getting it all done could be stressful.

There were times during my training for the 2004 Ironman Canada I wondered why I was doing it. There is a time commitment to this training that has a big impact on your family time. I felt guilty many times because of all the time I spent away from my girls. That was the most difficult aspect of all the training.

The human body is designed to move. I look back on my life with only one, big regret. It was the day I bought my first car. I thought it would bring me freedom. What it brought me was a dependence on something designed to make my life easier. We humans are conditioned to look for things to make life easier. I was still active after buying that car, by playing sports and enjoying other active pursuits, but it changed the mindset of my youth to that of a mindset of dependency.

Before I bought that car, I walked, ran or biked everywhere. Even in the cold, Canadian winters it was rare for me to ride the bus. It was even rarer to get rides from my parents (not like today). I walked or rode my bike to school all the time. When it was too cold to ride, then it meant I walked. That was just the way it was for me, and I can never recall feeling put out by that.

I work in the transportation industry. One thing I started to do early in my career was ride my bike or run to work. I would do it because I enjoyed those activities more than I did driving my vehicle. It was easy and NATURAL to run or ride my bike. I was not thinking environmentally or economically back in 1987. I was not even thinking; it was just pure joy that made me do this. I would even ride the bus to work and then run home after my shift. My mind would focus on the run as my means to exercise and be unique. There are a lot of unfit people who I have worked with over the years, and still do, in my industry. If being true is judgemental, then I guess I am being judgemental! The cost to society due to people who are unhealthy and unfit is huge.

There have been people I worked with who literally thought I was a freak. I didn't have the stereotypical attitude or mindset of the majority. I wasn't conforming to the ways of their world, so I was a freak and a target. I remember friends I worked with coming up and telling me how others truly thought I was a freak for running or riding to and from work! Some work mates would ask me, "Why would you do that?" My answer would be, "Why wouldn't I?" There is value in answering a question with a question when people think you are a freak. I just really enjoyed those activities more than sitting behind the wheel of a vehicle. It felt much more natural to run or ride my bike. I like being natural. I was following my true nature, my heart.

I have never done these things just to be different. Besides, if you want to spend all that money unnecessarily on gas and maintenance when there are other alternatives, then that is your business. However, if you want to think of me as a freak because I chose those alternatives, then I am fine with that. I am a freak—a freak that is fit, healthy, saving money and not a financial burden on the system.

I will not, however, condone a negative, aggressive or dangerous attitude of a driver towards cyclists. Driving is a privilege, not a right. Being a dangerous jerk is a choice. Luckily, I have never had any serious injuries because of motorists who just can't share the road with cyclists. I have had a few confrontations with aggressive and inconsiderate people behind the wheels of their cars. I would like to say that there are far more considerate drivers on the road than jerks. Many times drivers have been excellent stewards of safety and sharing the road, which is awesome. Thank you, drivers, for your consideration for us cyclists.

As for my fellow cyclists ... some of you can be jerks as well. Yes, you—the one who rides a block on the sidewalk, then is back out onto the road. And you—the one who goes through the red light. We have a responsibility to follow the rules of the road. I apologize to motorists for the jerk cyclists out there who cause issues for you.

I digress, though. Back to being a freak! When I analyze why I would do Ironman Canada, it really comes down to it being part of my true nature. I like a physical challenge and pushing myself in the physical realm. I have learned so much about myself from this type of challenge in my life. There is also a component of wisdom involved in why I would do it. The human body was not designed to be sedentary. Technology has stripped us of many natural actions our bodies were designed to perform and require to be healthy. I have always been in touch with that inner wisdom and felt drawn to be fit.

We minimize our Creator by allowing the body to deteriorate without need. Certainly there are circumstances that people can't control that can impact their health. God is capable of so many tremendous things that sometimes we only need to ask and act; He will take care of the rest. That body that you possess is capable of some extraordinary stuff.

I was designed for this type of physical activity; I feel it in my heart. In my journey, God brought me to physical challenges because He knew what purpose they would have for me. He understood the impact they would have on my life. My true nature would come to the surface because of these types of events.

Why would I do that? I would do it because I am passionate about what pulls me deeper in my relationship with God. In my training, racing and even thinking about something like Ironman, I find God. He is there in my space and time—coaching me, energizing me, and loving me.

I am a better person when I take the time to train. I am more focused and disciplined at those times. I am less frustrated and susceptible to depression. I find solutions to problems when I am out training. I feel alive and excited about the very life I have been blessed with. I am a freak for this type of stuff and, well, that makes me happy.

Chapter 15

Warrior Spirit

Endure the suffering along with me,
as a good soldier of Jesus Christ
(2 Timothy 2:3, NLT).

To start this chapter, I want to make it clear that I am not comparing myself to a soldier. Often we hear athletes, commentators and sports fans talk about their teams "going to battle." I have never felt comfortable comparing athletes, who often make millions of dollars playing a game, to soldiers in a war.

I have the utmost respect and admiration for the Canadian men and women serving this country in the military. That respect is extended to the men and women of the United States military, and to any allies of Canada. The sacrifices these individuals make for us, for little money and less recognition compared to athletes, should not be compared with what athletes do. There is no comparison. The value of our military personnel is greater than the contributions of athletes. I am a sports fan, but I find it harder every day to like what is taking place in many sports.

One of my favourite books is *Way of the Peaceful Warrior*[4] by Dan Millman. Millman relates the lessons he learned from the character Socrates in the book. At one point, Socrates explains to Millman how the mind is a construct of humans. The mind is not something tangible that can be pinpointed. Socrates explains that the brain is a tangible, physical thing that is real. I have found many great lessons in this book and have used it often as a means to try and grow as a person. The word "warrior" is broadly defined as a person engaged in some struggle or conflict. We are all warriors in some way, shape or form.

I have discovered that there are people who don't want anything difficult in their lives. If they can find the path of least resistance, they will choose it every time. These kinds of people complain any time things get tough, and they look for someone else to fix it for them, or to blame (I experienced a great deal of this in the union environment I worked in). I find this group of people have an unreal expectation of life. When anything happens that can upset the balance in their lives, they want it fixed now! They don't look for solutions; they look for the person with the solution. Often these people don't strive for excellence; instead, they settle for mediocrity and are apathetic in their lives and work (I work in an industry where the status quo rules the vast majority of the people in it).

It is easier for these people to not look at themselves and how their lack of drive, commitment, and work ethic impacts society and their employer. I so often hear and see these people blame the government, management and the rich for the state of affairs in society. They are adamantly set in their ways, and they are unwilling to change. I call these types of people the entitlement crowd.

Then there are the people I call warriors. These people don't expect anything from life, other than getting out of it what they put in. These are the people who are truly alive; they live each moment with passion. These people want to find the solutions and seek to help others see the benefits. When things need to be done, they roll their sleeves up and get after it. They are often people who seek little recognition for their efforts, but without them many things would never come to fruition. There is an inner energy that emanates from these warriors.

When things get tough and life creates challenges for the warriors, they just get tougher. Feeling sorry for themselves is not an option. To a warrior, that is energy wasted when it could be used for getting past whatever stands in their way. I have been blessed to work and play with some awesome warriors.

I am going to the word bank again. The word "indomitable" means to be incapable of being subdued. This is a character trait of the warrior. When you are training for an Ironman or other endurance events, this is a great quality to have. I have witnessed some people in life that have indomitable spirits. They just don't give up and will persevere through a lot to achieve their goals. There is tremendous discipline required for an indomitable spirit. People who break rules, laws and just don't care about their impact on others are not indomitable. They are selfish, irresponsible and care only about themselves. This is being undisciplined and reckless. I saw enough of these people in the union environment I worked in to know the difference between them and a warrior.

Warriors with an indomitable spirit are not willing to compromise their values and ethics. They don't want to get what they want at the expense of others without actually earning it. Incapable of being subdued, these individuals are willing to put forth the utmost effort and accept the consequences for their actions. Not to beat a dead horse, but in my past union work environment accountability was a joke, and the union promoted lack of accountability.

Earlier I mentioned the book *Be Unreasonable* by Paul Lemberg. The first chapter of that book is dedicated to what he defines as an "Unreasonable manifesto." The entire chapter is awesome, but here is an excerpt that I love:

> Being unreasonable requires rejecting compromises. Compromises force you to sacrifice what truly matters in exchange for efficiency and expediency. They are insubstantial things that exist because of a belief in a false context. Change the context and the compromise dissolves.[5] (Paul Lemberg)

I think that is brilliant! We compromise on everything in today's world. People take jobs, and then the employer has to compromise on things because of people's "rights." If the employer is changing things midstream and creating a dangerous workplace, then you have the right to opt out. But when you agree to a condition of employment that states you will wear a uniform, and then decide that it doesn't suit you, you are copping-out and going back on your word and your agreement.

We continually see compromise as a way to be amicable with each other. It is a way to avoid offending or upsetting people and keeping the status quo. I look around at society and ask: "How is all this compromising working for you?" Do not confuse your privileges with what you believe are your rights. They are totally different and compromise you more than you realize.

Warriors will not compromise on their actions, values or beliefs, because they want to achieve what they are doing. If I compromise on my training for an Ironman, who am I hurting? If I agree to a condition of employment then turn around and whine about it, what does that say about my character? Warriors don't see compromise as a win/win. It is allowing the seeds of dissent, ruin and failure to set in.

I discovered a part of myself while training for the Ironman Canada in 2004. I always knew I had a unique spirit, as we all do, but during that time I found the warrior within. I discovered that I have an indomitable spirit, and that I have always had it.

I once went to a professional for help preparing a resume. She talked with me about the difference between bragging and promoting myself. That was a real moment of enlightenment. I never used to talk about my accomplishments and successes, because I thought it was bragging. She convinced me to promote myself and be proud of what I had accomplished. The word "survivor" seems kind of drastic, but it is what I am. I survived a season in my life of shame, hate, anger and so much more that resulted from my abuse. It was not pretty or healthy at times for me or those around me, but ultimately I had to fight, scratch, work, hide, wait, run, punch, kick, scream and hope that one day I would get through to the other side.

I remember the days I didn't want to live anymore. I didn't want to hurt the people I loved with my black, dark moods and energy. I honestly thought that they and the world would be a better place without me. Life, at times, was not enjoyable for me, and there was that shame that hung over me like a tower of unimaginable weight and pain. At the same time, there was always something that kept me going, some small spark that would ignite my desires to get it together, some inspiration that made me look for another path that would bring me hope. I had faith that somehow it would all be fine. The day would come when I would experience the light, and my being would not be consumed in darkness forever.

Growing up Catholic, we went to church on Sundays because Dad believed in the value church would add to our lives. I remember loving it, though, when Sunday would roll around and we hit the church scene. I hung on every word when they spoke about Jesus. I could picture myself there beside Him as he walked and talked. It was a magical time for me as a boy. The faith I began with back then stuck somewhere deep down inside me. In the voice and inner presence of the Holy Spirit, that faith remained below the surface. Faith I didn't even understand I had and didn't practice would keep the warrior in me alive—that indomitable warrior that drove me to Ironman Canada was always present.

My inner warrior was a product of God's patience and coaching. All that I required to survive my darkest depths had been etched on my heart at birth, and slowly taught to me as I journeyed. I may have felt alone, but that was a choice. I was never alone. The deep love and mercy of God was continually wrapped around my heart, protecting me. His patience is infinite, and when I was ready, God stepped into my time and space to ensure I would succeed.

I believe Jesus was who he said he was—the Son of God. I believe that Jesus died on the cross for all mankind. I believe Jesus is my Saviour and will provide me with salvation. I believe Jesus was and is an incredible warrior who taught, lived, and created life.

I was called to compete in the 2004 Ironman Canada Triathlon for a reason. It would ultimately mark the end of a long season in my life. The warrior within me was being asked to trust my master. I was giving in to the will of God and the work Jesus began when He died for me. I was being healed as I journeyed toward this event. My mind and body were transformed as the Holy Spirit worked within me, setting me free from what I couldn't give up. I had a new way of looking at life that allowed me to experience my true nature, not the ways the world had formed in me.

Let me tell you how cool it is to experience freedom by training for and competing in Ironman Canada! This was not a tough task for me that had me cursing my decision. This was an awesome experience and pleasure for me. God knew me and what was going to heal me. Life is an adventure worth pursuing with passion and with every breath we take.

Chapter 16

Ironman Canada 2004

Sunday, August 28, 2004, started early for me. I set my alarm for 04:00. I woke up feeling well rested. On the Friday night before, I made sure to be in bed early and sleep long. I thought Saturday night would be a fitful sleep, but it wasn't. I slept well all through the night.

The sky was still dark with some daylight starting to creep across the morning sky. There appeared to be some cloud cover, but the weather forecast was for a nice sunny day. The day was finally here; my Ironman Canada dream was now upon me.

I was camping in a campground right in Penticton. It was located in a good, central area not far from the Start/Finish line, so there was not a lot of travel time to worry about. It had everything I required for my stay. I made my regular breakfast of scrambled eggs (a heaping helping) and enjoyed a cup of green tea. My friend, Shirley, from Canmore was with me for the race and was an immense help during the day and time leading up to Ironman. I am grateful to her for all her support and encouragement throughout my training. I made note of the fact that I was not feeling nervous about what lay ahead. More often than not before a race, I will be nervous. Today, I felt calm and confident. My mind was focused on this moment and what I needed to do in it to get myself fuelled up to start the race.

Over the previous two days, I had checked, rechecked, double checked and then checked all my gear again. I had dropped my bike off at the transition area on Saturday, where it stayed overnight. My swim to bike and bike to run transition bags had also been dropped off Saturday. I had my car packed with my special needs bags and everything I needed for the day. I was able to enjoy a nice breakfast without worrying and just relax. I was feeling focused.

Race start was at 07:00. I wanted to get to the start area early and make sure everything was in order. I drove through the quiet Penticton streets to a spot as close to the transition area as possible and parked. I was at the transition area just after 05:00, and there were already a lot of athletes there. I took my special needs bags for the run and bike to the drop off areas designated for them and left them there. Next, I went to the body marking station. Along with wearing a race bib, each athlete gets their race number marked on different areas of their bodies with a Sharpie. This is to help race officials and volunteers identify athletes on the course. Once I was done there, it was back to the transition area to check my run and bike transition bags one last time. Knowing that this was not necessary didn't stop me from doing it just to be sure. Then it was off to my bike to put air in the tires and do one last inspection of everything on it. It was ready and needed nothing else done to it.

I walked back to my car and rested inside for a few minutes. I went through my mental checklists and was satisfied everything was ready and in its place. I turned on my Ironman CD and closed my eyes to visualize my race. I was relaxed, and I focused on my breathing.

At 06:20 I entered the men's change tent in the transition area and started my final race preparations. I had my dry clothes bag with me to put my clothes in, so that at the end of the race I would have clothes to put on. I used my Body Glide (a lubricant that prevents chaffing and painful rubbing) on strategic areas of my body. I pulled on my wet suit and grabbed my swim goggles and the required swim cap.

I walked through the transition area and out onto the beach at 06:40. Lakeshore Drive was a mass of people who had come out to watch and cheer for family and friends who were racing. There were people along the beach retaining wall for a long, long way in both directions.

The beach was filling up with the more than 2500 athletes who would race Ironman. People were in the water warming up; some were making adjustments to their wetsuits or goggles and swim caps. Others talked nervously amongst themselves, or with people they knew who were standing along the retaining wall or in the water along the beach. I slid into the water for a quick warm-up and to get that initial cold water blast that takes my breath away each time out of the way. Confident that my wetsuit needed no adjustments, I walked back up to the beach and waited. There was a lot of white noise happening around me. The race announcer was making announcements over the P.A. system, and when he wasn't speaking there was music playing. There was a lot of noise from the athletes and spectators. It was all background noise to me; I was in my own world of mental focus and solitude. I was dialled in.

I was my own calm before the storm. I felt so peaceful in those moments before the race started. I closed my eyes, said a prayer of thanks, and asked God for strength to complete what I was about to do. I was feeling grateful and highly self-aware, waiting to begin the race I had prepared an entire year for.

The professional athletes begin the race earlier than the age group athletes. This way they do not get caught up in all the turbulence of the start and lose precious time. For these athletes, the race is about results that can mean making money or not. I watched them head out on their journey. The Canadian national anthem began to play, and I felt tears well up in my eyes. I am proud and blessed to be Canadian, and the emotion was strong as I was standing there listening. Once the anthem was done, we had a minute to wait before the race would start.

The race announcer started to count down the final seconds. Ten, nine, eight … this is it, I thought! Seven, six, five, four … relax and don't go out to fast; pace yourself! Three, two, one… BOOM! An air horn was blasted and the world around me went silent.

The swim start of an open water triathlon can be a rough place. Bodies are running into the water as deeply as they can. Then arms start to flail and feet begin to kick. Bad things can happen with over 2500 people all rushing in to swim. Goggles can get dislodged, people get accidently punched, and it can be chaos. I was fortunate and didn't encounter any bad stuff during the swim start. Even with all the chaos going on around me, I felt calm. I found my pace and rhythm quickly. I felt comfortable in the water and was glad to have the race underway.

The swim course is a weird sort of triangular shape. The first leg is 1612 metres long; the course is marked by orange buoys on the athletes' right side. After a right turn at a big houseboat, the second leg is then 450 metres long. Athletes turn right again and onto the final leg, which is 1800 metres long.

I am not an exceptionally fast swimmer, so I exited the 2.4 mile swim course in one hour and twenty two minutes. The swim went well and, thankfully, uneventfully. I was happy and feeling good as I ran up towards the transition area to have my wetsuit stripped off (there are strippers at Ironman who peel your wetsuit off for you). The athlete takes their arms out of their wetsuit and pulls the top portion down to their waist. Once they get to the grassy area of the transition area, they lie on their backs and two strippers yank on the wetsuit arms, stripping it off—hence the name "strippers."

I didn't rush once I was in the tent. I took my time to ensure I dried off and was able to pull my bike shorts and cycling jersey on without any struggle. I wanted the 112 mile bike ride to start out on a comfortable note. What happened after that was not something I could control completely, but this I could.

I spent over ten minutes in the swim to bike transition, which is a long time. I didn't worry about the time as much as ensuring I was comfortable and prepared to get on the bike. I walked out of the tent to my bike and grabbed it. Then I walked to the mount/dismount line on the pavement, climbed on and started to ride.

The bike course takes athletes onto Main Street, which is lined on either side with spectators. It was an incredible feeling riding down Main Street and seeing all the people out there cheering for us. It was inspiring and energizing to hear the clapping and cheering.

"Way cool," I thought to myself.

It didn't take long to get down Main Street and past all of those people. After a few quick turns, the course heads out Eastside Road at the south end of Penticton. It takes you along the shore of Skaha Lake, which has a lot of great scenery to take in. I settled into a rhythm and tried not to go too fast with all the other cyclists around me. When people passed me, I wanted to make sure not to get caught up in their pace and go too fast. It required a lot of focus and patience to not overextend myself.

One of my goals for this Ironman was to make sure I enjoyed myself and the experience. I had a time goal that I was aiming to complete the race in. The main goal was to finish this race, so I needed to be wise. I wanted to make sure I enjoyed it all, as there is a lot to take in during the event.

On the bike course, there were aid stations every twenty kilometres or so. The aid stations had Gatorade, water, energy gels and fruit that athletes could replenish themselves with as they rode. My nutrition plan consisted of drinking Gatorade and water, eating hard boiled eggs and almonds, and using energy gels. I love eggs and find them to be the protein for me, so I carried the eggs and almonds with me. Ironman racing requires taking in food and energy because of the distance and time elements of the race. Proper nutrition while racing can mean the difference between a great race and a horror story. I was confident with my nutrition plan, and had used it during the 2004 Great White North Half Ironman in July as a test (and I didn't fall off my bike this time).

After the first hour in the saddle, I popped my first hardboiled egg and ate it. I was going to eat an egg every hour on the bike, and mix in some almonds here and there. The first egg tasted awesome, and I felt good getting some food on board. I was riding well, drinking water and eating some gels, too.

After the second hour, I ate my second hardboiled egg, but it didn't digest that well. I had to chew a lot more than usual and drink water to get it digested. I was burping a lot for some reason after eating it, which was weird. I worried a little bit about it, but didn't give it too much energy and remained calm mentally.

After my third hour, eating the hardboiled egg did not go so well. I had only tried to eat half the egg and I felt like I was going to puke. No amount of Gatorade or water was helping to wash it down; it only made me feel worse. I didn't even try to eat the second half of the egg, because I didn't want to throw up. What the heck was going on? I tried to eat some almonds to see if the result would be any different. I only tried to eat four, but that was not a successful experiment. I had to wash them down with water, because I was struggling to swallow them. Now I was full on worried. This was not something I had anticipated, and I was kind of freaked out.

I continued to drink Gatorade and eat gels. At the fifth aid station, I grabbed a banana. I literally had to force the banana down and chase it with water to swallow it. I was feeling bad just trying to keep the banana down. What was going on, man?

I was still riding at my pace, but physically I was starting to feel less and less energy. I was glad to be able to at least take in the energy gels as I rode. Mentally I was worried; I knew what not getting enough food into me could mean in this race. I was over half way in the bike portion of the race, but still had a long way to go. I wondered if I would BONK (physically run out of energy, suck, hurt ... BONK!).

Over the next hour I would get my answer. There is an out and back section on the bike course. At this point, you turn back on a different road and ride in the direction from which you came. It means going in the opposite direction of where you will need to go to finish the bike course. By the time I turned out and headed away on this section of the course, I was a hurting unit. I had no energy and was trying to get through on gels and Gatorade. For the first time on this journey, I had some doubts about finishing this thing! How was I going to finish without eating? This was not going well.

Dave, my coach, had given me some advice a few weeks before Ironman that popped into my vacant, worried mind. He had said, "Think your way through it. Ironman is a long race. Am I going too fast? Am I eating enough, or too much? Think your way through it."

I needed to calm and focus my mind. I made a decision to slow down my pace. If I conserved energy, I had some stuff in my special needs bag that may help. I focused on the out and back turnaround and didn't think about anything else. Every ten minutes I ate an almond or two, if I could force them down, just to get something solid into me.

When I reached the special needs area on the bike course, after the turnaround, a volunteer handed me my special needs bag. All athletes have the option of preparing a bag for this location, which is trucked out for them to this spot. I had jujubes, more almonds and gels in my bag. I pulled over a couple of hundred feet from the bag area, got off my bike, and sat down. I ate a handful of the jujubes and waited to see what would happen. After a couple of minutes I wasn't feeling like puking them up, so I ate another handful. I grabbed a handful of almonds and chewed them up well and swallowed. Another minute later I still felt nothing. Awesome! I had some solid food in my gut. Jujubes are not nutritional in any way, but at that moment they were manna from heaven.

Another competitor was sitting about ten yards from me. He was getting ready to start riding again. He looked at me and asked if I wanted the last half of the 500 ml Coke he had been drinking; he didn't want any more. I gladly accepted the bottle. I drank the first gulp and swallowed; it was so refreshing. I drank the bottle down and got ready to push on.

I had been off the bike for over ten minutes. It would impact my overall time, but I wasn't worried about that. As I got back to riding, I had a renewed sense of energy. Physically, I was able to ride my pace without too much effort. Mentally, I was feeling refreshed, and my confidence was back.

Things went well for me until a place on the bike course called Yellow Lake Road. It is just before you hit the century point of the ride, which is at one hundred miles. The last big hill of the ride is at this point, and it is fairly steep. It's the last big test on the bike; once up this hill, I knew I would get this ride done. However, I had to get up the hill first! Easier said than done, Daniel! I had been eating jujubes, almonds and gels, which had given me energy to get to this point. When I got to the bottom of Yellow Lake, I wasn't doing too badly. As the road pitched up and I needed more effort, I found I wasn't feeling it. I turned the pedals over slowly and deliberately as I started to ascend a hill that seemed insurmountable as I started to climb it. At points going up that hill I felt like I was crawling. At the three quarter point, I didn't know if I could do it. I looked at the bracelets Shayla and Aislinn made and focused on each pedal stroke. I had to get up that hill.

Yellow Lake is a popular spot for spectators to come out and watch the race. They write chalk messages on the hill to spur on their friends or loved ones racing. I was getting constant encouragement from the people who were standing along the roadside. It gave me energy to keep painfully turning my legs over to keep moving. There can be a lot of traffic on the road at this point of the race. People are leaving to get back to town and see their racers heading off on the run. I was slowly making my way up the hill alongside cars that were not moving quickly due to the volume of traffic on the road. To my left in the traffic was a yellow Mustang convertible with four young men in it. It would move up a couple lengths and then have to stop. I would ride slowly up the hill and catch up to them while they were stopped. One young dude yelled over to me as I rode up beside them.

"Look at you, man. You're passing a Mustang; you're so fast. You're going to be an Ironman, buddy."

I had to laugh and it made me smile. All I could muster was to turn and smile at these guys, giving them thumbs up. They all gave me the thumbs up back and hooted and hollered. That was what I needed. They had made me feel good, and I was almost at the top of the hill. I was going to get up that hill. Yeah!

After the steep part of Yellow Lake there are a couple of shorter, less steep sections near the top, but they are gradual inclines. Once past them it is mostly downhill into Penticton. My mental energy and mindset switched completely now. I was buoyed by the thought that I would soon be back in Penticton, headed to transition area. The downhill portion of the highway leading into Penticton was so wonderful. A mental lightness filled me, and I enjoyed the scenery of Skaha Lake and the surrounding countryside. Once back in Penticton, it was a short ride down Main Street to transition. At one point, you pass the area where runners are turning off Main Street to head out to Eastside Road on the run. It was cool thinking I would soon be running back this way.

People lined Main Street, still cheering and watching. I was once again filled with energy at the cheers and encouragement. I turned off Main Street and rode the final two hundred metres to the bike dismount line. I stopped at the line on the pavement and got off my bike. A volunteer took my bike from me and placed it back in my spot. I love my bike; however, I didn't want to see it again for a month! I walked to the change tent to get my run gear on and go for a short run (this was a mental joke I used to lighten the mood for the marathon I now faced). A feeling came over me in that moment; I was going to do this, even with how bad I felt at times on the bike. I now felt completely sure that I would finish this race. I was not being over confident; I just felt in my gut it was going to happen. I felt that heart energy rise up, and I was smiling a smile like never before.

I changed into my running gear, taking my time to ensure I was prepared for the marathon ahead. I chatted with a few other athletes and some volunteers in the tent. I felt calm and at ease about what was ahead. It was amazing how my mental and physical energies had shifted over the final twenty kilometres of the bike course. Now I was energized and positive about what I was doing.

Dave had told me about the aid stations on the run having chicken soup broth. I laughed when he first told me this, thinking it was rather strange. As I was leaving the bike to run transition, I stopped at the aid station, grabbed a cup of soup broth and sipped it slowly. The salt tasted so good! I swear I could feel my body absorbing the salt. It was rejuvenating me so much. I felt fresh and strong.

I headed out for the run feeling quite renewed and oh so alive. *I am doing this Ironman*, I told myself. *I am now 26.2 miles from crossing that finish line. Focus and pace, Daniel, that will get you there. You will be an Ironman.*

The run heads out on Main Street for a block then turns to the west on Westminster Avenue and heads down to Winnipeg Street. Once there, athletes turn north and head to Lakeshore Drive and run west along Lakeshore, which takes them back along Okanogan beach. A kilometre after running west, they turn around and head back east on Lakeshore again. Then it is back onto Winnipeg Street and down to Westminster and east to Main Street, where they now run south. The run follows Main Street then heads out along east side road, which runs parallel to Skaha Lake. The athletes follow this road until it enters the community of OK Falls, which is the half-way point of the marathon run. Here, they turn around and retrace their steps back to Penticton.

Ironman Canada provides athletes with two race bibs for the event. One has your number and first name on it, and the second has your number and last name on it. When on the run course, you are required to have the bib number facing forward for officials and volunteers to see. I wore my bib with my first name on it during the run. As I ran, spectators kept yelling out encouragement like, "Go Daniel," "Awesome effort, Daniel; you look great," and so on. It was truly invigorating and awesome to get that support from people.

As an "age group" athlete at Ironman, you feel like a professional. We race the same course as the pros, and there are spectators and supporters all over the course. Running along Lakeshore and then back out of town along Main Street is an experience I will never forget. The energy you get from the people along the course is an awesome and magical experience. When athletes get out along Eastside Road many residents come out and offer support as well. This section of the run is beautiful, and there were many encounters with people along it that were fun. People would joke with me, and I would make wise cracks to them about wanting the beer they had in their hands. It helped to keep the mind off the distance ahead, and to bring levity to the situation.

Runners heading out of town see runners coming back into town on their way to the finish line. There are aid stations every mile along the run course where athletes can take on fuel and get water. I was not feeling bad at the start of the run and was keeping up a pretty good pace. I made sure to fuel as much as possible at each aid station along the way. When you get close to the turnaround at OK Falls, there are a few hills to climb before you go down one big hill. It is about the seventeen or eighteen kilometre point on the run. By this time, I was starting to feel tired. Trying to run after walking through the aid stations was becoming harder each time. Soon the walking was longer than the running.

I went through a mental checklist to take stock of where I was at. I wasn't hurting in any way at all. I was just tired. I was able to run down the long hill into OK Falls and to the turnaround, where I got my special needs run bag. I had jujubes in there, which I was glad to eat quickly. I also had a couple of gels I took with me, just in case I needed them.

After the short time in OK Falls it was time to retrace my steps back to Penticton and the finish line. Now I was faced with the daunting task of getting myself back up the hill I had run down. It was much easier running down than going back up. I tried to run, but it was just not going to happen, so I conserved energy and walked. I find that the mind will quit much quicker than the body will give in. One of the reasons I push myself is to overcome the limitations of my mind. I want to one day not have any trouble mentally in a race like Ironman and not give in. That day was not the day, however, but it didn't have an impact on my energy. From the turnaround at OK Falls back to the city limits of Penticton, I did more walking than running. At times I tried to force myself to run and go for one hundred metres or so before I had to stop and walk. My legs just didn't have any power left in them.

I enjoyed the experience, though, and just made sure to keep smiling and looking at the scenery along Skaha Lake. I focused on each kilometre along the stretch and counted down how many kilometres I had left after passing each kilometre marker. Entering back into Penticton at kilometre thirty six, I was struck by an awesome insight. It was simple in its nature and reality, but for me it meant an incredible amount. In only six kilometres, I would be crossing the Ironman Canada finish line! It seemed like an eternity ago that the race had begun, and like a lifetime ago that I had signed up. Now here I was moving continually towards that line—the place I said I was going to cross no matter what.

I was walking along and saw an ambulance ahead of me pulled over with its lights on. As I walked closer, I noticed an athlete sitting in the back with a couple of paramedics and a race official there. When I was within ear shot, I heard the athlete pleading that he was alright to continue. One of the paramedics told him that his blood pressure was too high and they couldn't allow him to continue. What a drag, I thought. I felt so bad for the guy that I wanted to jump into the ambulance and spring him so he could finish the race. I wondered if this was his first race, or had he done this before? To be so close to the end and have it end this way would certainly be a hard pill to swallow. How harsh a reality for that athlete! But that is the reality of Ironman. All athletes know when they enter that if something medical comes up and it is serious, you will not be allowed to continue. And there would be no consolation medal or participation ribbon for that athlete at the end of the race, just a DNF (did not finish) next to his name in the results.

Unlike so many things in life where we give people an out and coddle them, Ironman Triathlon is an absolute. You have to do the distance in the allotted time. It may seem harsh, but when you sign up for it that is a reality you face. It is part of the challenge and lure that makes this race so amazing.

I quickly turned my attention back to myself and focused on me. I still had work to do here, I told myself as I settled back into my walking rhythm. I had come this far; I didn't want to allow anything to come between me and that finish line. Focus on that next kilometre marker and get to it!

The crowds of spectators grew larger along Main Street as I continuously moved from kilometre marker to kilometre marker. The energy around me grew more vibrant with each step I took. This created an inner energy that started to carry me quicker in my pace towards that line. As I moved further north along Main Street, I could hear the race announcer more clearly. When the race announcer wasn't talking, there would be fast paced music playing, which was nice to hear. People were everywhere along the street, cheering and yelling for athletes making their way to that line.

I retraced my steps west on Westminster Ave then north on Winnipeg Street. I made the turn away from the finish line to go west on Lakeshore Drive, which was cruel after such a long distance. Then I made it to the turnaround point on Lakeshore Drive and headed back towards the finish line. My legs found the energy to run; it wasn't fast, but it was running. I could see the powerful lights run by generators down near the Penticton Lakeside Resort Hotel and just kept running along as steady as I could. I was almost there; that line was beckoning to me.

I looked down at the bracelets around my wrist and thought about Shayla and Aislinn. I felt an emotional wave rise up in my heart as I thought about them. I hoped that by doing this it would set an example for them in some way that they could emulate in their lives. Part of me wondered if I was teaching them a good lesson, or if this was just a selfish pursuit. I wished they were there at that moment to share this with me.

As I approached the last two hundred metres, I thought about the race in terms of being one of my greatest accomplishments. The sides of Lakeshore Drive were lined with people cheering and giving me high fives. The noise was loud and pulling me along toward that line that was now towering ahead of me under the Ironman Race arch finish. As I reached the final hundred metres and got onto the red carpet leading to that line, it didn't feel like I was running anymore. I felt like I was riding a wave of energy. I wasn't tired anymore. I felt so refreshed and alive in that moment as I approached the tape stretched across the line by two volunteers.

I broke across the tape and the race announcer said, "Daniel O'Neill—you are an Ironman!" I wanted to show respect for this race and this moment. I had thought about how I would mark the end of this journey when I crossed the finish line. I placed my left hand palm down on top of my right hand made into a fist and bowed. This was how we entered the Temple in Kung Fu and was a sign of respect.

The Ironman medal was placed around my neck, and a volunteer approached me quickly to see how I was doing. She put an emergency blanket around my shoulders and asked me a few questions. I was feeling well and was in no need of medical attention. We walked to the table where I was given my finisher hat and t-shirt. The volunteer lady walked me to the change tent and left me in the hands of a male volunteer. I changed into my dry clothes and gathered up my bags and bike. This was after I sat quietly in the tent for a bit to savour the moment and reflect on what I had just done.

My friend, Shirley, was there waiting for me, and she drove me back to the campground. I didn't unload the stuff from the car because I just wanted to get to the shower and clean off. Standing in that shower for about ten minutes felt so good and cleansing. I was hungry, but it was the last thing on my mind, and I didn't really want to expend the energy on trying to eat. I made my way back to the tent and lied down with a sigh on the bed. It felt so good just lying there. I thought about what I had just done, and don't think it had truly sunk in yet. It was quiet in the campground, and I enjoyed the stillness of the night and myself. I said a prayer of thanks to my Creator for everything and for getting me here. I drifted off to sleep with the thought that I was now an Ironman.

Having done this event since 2004, and being there many times to witness it, I am amazed at what it takes to get this done. There are professionals who will do this Ironman in less than eight and a half hours. That type of effort and accomplishment is mind boggling.

There are people who will finish this event in just under the seventeen hour allotted time. That too is an amazing accomplishment. Then there are all the people in between who finish and can put the Ironman Canada check mark on their resume. Each and every person who does it is truly an amazing individual.

I love to watch the Ironman, whether as a participant or a spectator. I love it because it is a test of the human will and desire. We are designed to move, to challenge, and to accomplish all that the Creator instilled within us as His children. God loves watching us attempt to reach higher levels of life by pursuing the things that celebrate the creations we are.

I am not only talking about Ironman here, but every time a human pushes themselves past their comfort zone to achieve something. It could be running your first ten kilometre race. It may be learning how to swim, bike or skate. It may be creating by doing needlepoint or painting. It is all about being a part of the human being experience and pleasing the Lord.

Completing this Ironman was a part of my healing journey. God took me to a place He knew would help me move past the things that were blocking my ability to be me. I found an inner energy to help me create a new perspective on who I am and where I fit in the world.

The joy and peace I would experience and that would grow in me from this entire journey was so welcomed by me. I had returned to relationship with my Creator, and I was happy that I had been given the opportunity to explore that relationship in such a truly wonderful and challenging fashion.

Chapter 17

Life is an Endurance Event

"...and let us run with endurance
the race God has set before us."
(Romans 12:1b, NLT)

I SLEPT FOR ABOUT SEVEN HOURS BEFORE I WOKE UP ON MONDAY, August 29, 2004. My tent was warm, and I had slept so well throughout the night. The real test was about to come, as I had to try and get out of bed. I was surprised to find out that I was not stupid sore as I got up! Walking was not even really painful, and that was nice. I had to get some food, as I was starving. A big breakfast of bacon, eggs, hash browns and toast seemed like it was the best meal I had ever eaten. The food tasted so good, and I savoured every bite. It was good enough to fill me up for now, which was the purpose.

I walked around the Ironman expo and checked out the finisher swag. I met with friends and we all discussed our Ironman stories and adventures. Athletes were walking around in their finisher shirts and hats. It was enjoyable being there in the moment to see people happy with what they had accomplished.

I have stated that Ironman has absolute cut off times for each discipline in the race. If you don't make it to the end of each discipline before the cut off time, they don't allow you to go on. You could cross the finish line at one minute after midnight, which would mean missing the seventeen hour cut off. You would not become an Ironman. It sounds cruel, but that is Ironman, and competitors know it going in (I wish the politically correct ways of this world would recognize the benefits of this for the people who are being enabled in society).

It may seem weird to believe that God would take me to Ironman Canada to bring me back into relationship with Him, but the universe has a design to it and it was designed by the Creator, God. I was brought to this place on earth in this time to help me understand all the lessons God had created for me to this point in my life. This one year journey and season in my life was orchestrated by God to help me understand my place in the circle. It was intended to show me my true nature, instilled in me by God. I was healed of a past that was out of my control. God allowed me the freedom to heal in a way that meant so much to me.

I speak of God entering my space and time. By this I mean that God physically walked with me and guided me. God touched my heart and opened it to His presence and the peace of His energy bestowed on me by His grace. I do not claim to be an expert in all things pertaining to God; I am just a lucky dude who was allowed to explore who I am in a truly cool way. My Creator presented me with an opportunity to understand that all my life's pursuits had been designed to bring me closer and closer to Him. When God knew I was ready and needed Him most, He opened my eyes with Ironman Canada. God understands me so well that He understood that this race and the required training would bring me into relationship with Him.

God walks into our lives, space and time in a personal and physical way. We are waves of energy that He created in a unique way that makes us like no other human being. God knows us intimately in ways we don't even know ourselves. When we believe we are alone, He works in the shadows, creating for us. At the end of my favourite movie, *Vision Quest*, Louden Swain achieves his goal. It is a goal that people think is unattainable, crazy and impossible—but he does it. Swain says this about the journey to his goal:

> But all I ever settled for is that we're born to live and then to die, and ... we got to do it alone, each in his own way. And

I guess that's why we got to love those people who deserve it like there's no tomorrow. 'Cause when you get right down to it—there isn't.[6]

I use to believe that, wanted to believe that, and actually needed to believe that. In our humanity we are alone, but within our spirit we have the guide who created us; we walk with God.

My Ironman Canada journey was a season in my life from July 2003 to August 2004. This season would create changes in me I never would have created on my own. God pushed me to a new level of energy and higher awareness. I was a changed man, renewed by God like He promised in Romans 12:2.

You know what is funny? God asked me to obey Him and make sacrifices for Him, so Ironman became a test for me. It was a chance to have faith in and obedience to my Creator. What a terrible sacrifice to have to make, eh? What it turned out to be was a beautiful gift from my Creator, who allowed me to sacrifice in such a meaningful and powerful way. God knew what this would do for me.

I discovered something along the way to Ironman that I had not experienced in a long time—joy! Things in my life had been a chore, many a burden, and a plight I had to deal with. I had little meaning in my life, or hope for where I was going. This journey had changed and altered my perception of life. I hadn't liked myself very much for a long, long time. I felt I was not useful or important, because of the work I did. Life was not something I lived; it was something I had to do. I believed I had no choice. What had I done that was worthwhile? Not much, I thought. I was low on self-esteem and had no self-worth. Ironman training, racing and living brought me joy. I felt that incredible heart energy surging through my body and elevating me to new heights. The world of societal pressure, conditioning and conformity had been lifted. My inner balance had been restored. It felt good to be Daniel, and good to be alive.

Sometimes the word "purpose" is overused in life. I think intentional living is better than having a purpose alone. I like to think God has a purpose for all of us. I highly recommend *The Purpose Driven Life* [7] by

Rick Warren. It was brought into my life on this journey, and it helped me immensely along the way. It is our mission in life to intentionally fulfill God's mission for us. Many times we create a purpose that is counterproductive to what God created us for. Often we are our own worst enemies and follow the societal conditioning over our truth.

During my Ironman journey, I discovered how I had been cheating myself. I had been settling for mediocrity as the measuring point for my life. All my negativity and pessimism had been creating a man without hope. I had fallen ill in mind and body, but never in spirit. I had only lost touch with my spirit and the wisdom of my Creator contained therein. There are no ordinary moments in life; there is just ordinary societal conditioning. We have far greater capacity within us than we take the time to get into and cultivate. Each moment we walk in this gift called life is far from ordinary.

You and I are not ordinary; we are extraordinary human beings. No two people have, or will be, the same. The energy of which we are composed is uniquely different than that of anyone else. Each human being is created to be a unique, one of a kind, priceless being. Yet we are often taught to mould or pattern ourselves after other people. In God's eyes, you are a masterpiece built to be a precise, amazing piece of art in His creation. In that creation He has given you a unique art form that no other person can perform in God's great and infinite plan. In God's eyes, none of us is greater than or less than the other. We are all equal in our Creator's eyes.

Your position in life does not dictate your mission; your education, or lack of one, does not dictate your mission. How big, small, fit, healthy or mature you are doesn't dictate it, either. God dictates your mission, and He will create everything required to fulfill it. You only need to walk it through. In the quiet, still and peaceful heart God gave us all is where your mission is written. Your mind does not have the capacity to fathom what God created in you. The mind is too busy; it wants to control you and your environment. Silence is a place within you where all your energy is waiting for the Lord to direct it.

Life is an endurance event. It can be difficult, painful, and hard to deal with at times. The tests we experience can push us to the edge and make us want to quit. We will fail many times along the path we are asked to walk. Failure is just another opportunity to try. Not trying is more harmful than trying and failing. Life is not always fair, but man is it awesome.

God will ask you to journey in your own way. During this particular season, He asked me to follow the Ironman goal and commit to it. It was also during this season that God asked me to write this book. I have struggled a long time with this book. I have written and then re-written it five times. I have quit at times and vowed to never start again. I use to have hair when I started writing this thing, but not anymore. Just like Ironman in 2004 was a process I had to go through, and by which God transformed me, writing this book has taught me to trust God and find in Him these words and ideas. I am not a completed project yet, and I have much still to learn and understand. It is my hope that I will never be a completed project, because then life may become boring again.

As a Christian, I am not telling you how to live or that I know what is best for you. I am relaying my experience at Ironman Canada in 2004. It is about how God entered and walked with me in my space and time. I believe He is looking to walk with you as well. God created you and He loves you unconditionally. He wants to be in relationship with you like you are with your family and friends.

Each of us will be called in our own way. Was my calling glamorous? Well, maybe not to you. It is not about our societal view of important, glamorous and cool. It is about God's mission for each of us. It is about the importance that each of us has in His master plan. I think the way God brought me back into relationship with Him and healed me is ULTRA COOL!

You were designed to endure this race you now run. It may seem long and difficult; however, you are not alone. You will never be alone. Ask God for help; there is no special way or specific time you have to do it. Open your heart and let Him walk in. God will create what is necessary for you to succeed. Drop the conditioning of our world, and the truth will fill you with abundance.

Nobody Can Take It Away From You

A MONTH AFTER I HAD REACHED MY GOAL AND COMPLETED MY FIRST Ironman Canada in 2004, I was feeling a little down. For more than a year my energy had been directed towards achieving that one goal. I lived and breathed almost every moment in pursuit of it. From July of 2003 until August 28, 2004, I was consumed by a journey and lived it. After returning home and resuming the normalcy of my life without the goal I had been so passionate about for a year, I felt lost. All the time, energy and training had been worth it, and I had succeeded. Now what, though? I felt empty without the pursuit to keep me occupied, like a part of me had been removed. I did a few runs and gentle bike rides, but they weren't the same.

I needed to get a few new tubes for my bike tires, so I went to my favourite triathlon shop, Way Past Fast. The owner knew I had done Ironman that year and asked me how it went. I told him I had finished it in a respectable time, and that it was an amazing experience. I expressed I was a little disappointed because I hadn't achieved the time goal I had set for the race, and he said, "No one can take it away from you."

BOOM! WOW! Those eight words struck me like a lightning bolt! Those words reached into my heart and stoked that inner energy fire. How simple a phrase it was: "No one can take it away from you." Yet it was so profound in that moment. I bought my tire tubes and walked out of the store in a bit of a haze. The profound nature of those words was not just found in that moment alone. "No one can take it away from you" summed up the whole one year journey to Ironman. It summed up my return to relationship with God. It summed up my life to that point, and how I had come to be an Ironman.

No matter what happens in your life, relationship with God will carry you through. People, society, work, culture and so many other things will impact you, but no matter what happens to you, God will be there for you in your space and time if you allow Him to be. God has never and will never forsake us. I tried so hard to run away and be angry with God. I felt I was entitled to feel what I did because of my youth. God just patiently waited for the right time to fully show Himself to me. All through the days when I was unfaithful to Him, He was preparing the way for me. God held me close, and I was not even aware of how much He did for me. His Word says, *"God himself has prepared us for this, and as a guarantee he has given us his Holy Spirit"* (2 Corinthians 5:5, NLT).

"No one can take it away from you." What I thought had been lost was not lost at all. The beautiful gift of the Holy Spirit had been with me forever. Nothing can take that away from me, or from you if you are open to it. It is a truly wonderful way to live; it is real and rational to have a relationship with God.

I use the scriptures in a way that works for me. What you read, how you use them, and what they teach you may be different. I am not an expert on the Bible, or its factual and historical accuracy. It is a choice I make to believe that God is speaking to us through His word, and that the wisdom contained in that Word is timeless and will lead any one through their lives, no matter what day or age.

I am not big on religion, as anything can be turned into religion. I could say it is my religion to push my body to extreme lengths to determine what I am made of. It is more important for me to find the voice of God in myself while out trying to see what I am made of. I enjoy going to church, but I enjoy going out into the church of my environment and living the inner feelings of my spirit. What do I mean by hearing the voice of God? Pretty crazy, I guess, if you can't get past the surface of your conditioned human conformity. I prefer to be a human being than a human critically thinking and having to impose my will on the world because I am insecure and need to be right.

Being a human means making mistakes and not always getting it right. I have failed often at endurance events and felt bad. That feeling soon passes when I realize how grateful I am to have the ability, opportunity and mindset to try. I encourage you to find your challenge in life and pursue it. Allow the voice of God to enter your heart and guide you. It is really a cool thing to walk with Him. The voice I hear is distinct. It would move me at one point two years after Ironman in 2004 to leave a dead end job. The voice spoke these words clearly to me, "What are you doing here?" I knew instantly that God was challenging me to move out of my apathetic mode of survival and trust Him.

Two days later, I walked into my supervisor's office and gave notice I was leaving my job. I had no plan or back up job to go to, and I had two kids to support. Talk about crazy! In His amazing way, however, God created a job opportunity for me within one week. I got to work in a private company with a great business owner named Scott. It was an awesome experience, and I learned an awful lot from Scott that has helped me grow as a person. I will be blunt and honest here. I was so happy to be out of a unionized work environment, where entitlement and apathy were just the everyday norm. I am not a fan of the union mentality. I am not anti-union, but I believe they need to change. It's demoralizing working with people who do not perform and who continually don't follow their conditions of employment, but never get let go because of an archaic system. Enough said. I was out and life would never be the same. I am far better off now than I was staying in the security of a prison of apathy. Once again, God moved me and the end result was simply amazing. Yup, I am crazy in love with that voice and want to hear it as much as possible. I will note I have worked with many great people and know others who are in unions and are individuals with great character. It is not my intention to paint all union workers with the same brush.

I have struggled with the pride I have felt in calling myself an Ironman. I am proud of the fact I was able to swim 2.4 miles, bike 112 miles and then run 26.2 miles. It is not an easy thing to accomplish and requires a tough mindset and work ethic, so I feel proud of doing what I did (and have now done three times). I had the Ironman Canada logo tattooed on my right leg twice, because both times I did the race (in 2004 and 2008) it marked an incredible point of growth and change in my life. I fought through adversity in both years to finish an incredible race. "Nobody can take it away from you!" I am proud to be an Ironman and part of that fraternity of people who challenge the realm of possibility and are humans being.

I have a Nike swoosh tattooed on my left leg just above the ankle (I am asking for trouble because I never asked Ironman or Nike for permission to use their logos. Please forgive me if you can, guys.) Why? Because Nike was a company that inspired me many times when I was not feeling inspired. Their motto, "Just Do It," sums up what I feel like when I undertake a challenge. There is a spirit about an organization that pushes the envelope to move people. Whether you like Nike or not is of course up to you. Personally, I think without Nike there would be many more unhealthy people in our society from a lack of desire and motivation. "Nobody can take it away from you." The connection between the spirit of Nike and my spirit ignited a man to move when he was not feeling like it at all. The vision of Nike allowed me to see hope in a time when I felt no hope for me at all. I am thankful to Nike for their vision.

I am a simple man; my vision has driven me to the levels of my achievement and pushed me beyond what I imagined myself capable of at times. I am never going to win an Ironman. I am usually in the lower half of the finisher's results, but at Ironman that doesn't matter. The last finisher at an Ironman race is usually one of the most celebrated athletes of the day. Ironman creates heroes in everyone who tries, simply because they try. There is energy and magic at an Ironman that words cannot describe. You simply have to attend one to understand the meaning of the race. The Ironman Canada race is so emotionally charged with the human spirit it just sweeps you up and makes you want to live; there are no ordinary moments at Ironman.

After that first Ironman was completed in 2004, I couldn't help but wonder where God would lead me now. I hoped there would be more physical challenges like the one I was just able to complete, and there have been. I would gladly walk through another one like it with God as my coach. "No one can take it away from you."

There is an excellent Zen saying which states, "In the beginner's mind there are many possibilities. In the expert's mind there are few" (Shunryu Suzuki).[8]

I want to remain a beginner for the rest of my life. In my relationship with God, I want to keep an open mind, not one that is closed because I believe I know so much. In all areas of my life I want to remain a beginner, because the Daniel that isn't in that mindset can be closed minded. I keep reminding myself about the above saying and then add, "No one can take it away from you."

I learned during my Ironman journey in 2004 to be more childlike and live life. I don't need to be in control, which will only create more pressure. I can roll with life, and when bad things happen there is an inner guide who will willingly help me find solutions or ways to stick it out. When things are going well, it is fun to spread the energy and try to help others feel that power. "Nobody can take it away from you."

It is a beautiful thing to rediscover who you were born as and who you were born to be. To see a clear vision of yourself that you can work towards and strive to be is exhilarating. Life is an amazing journey filled with adventure; it has no better reward than walking it with your Creator. His love for us is all encompassing, eternal and unconditional. "No one can take it away from you." Not even the conditioning and ways of this world.

Endnotes

1. Paul Lemberg, *Be Unreasonable: The Unconventional Way to Extraordinary Business Results* (New York, N.Y., McGraw-Hill Education, 2007).

2. Bruce H. Lipton, *The Biology of Belief: Unleashing the Power of Consciousness, Matter and Miracles* (India, Hay House, 2008).

3. Dr. Wayne Dyer, *The Power of Intention* (India, Hay House, 2004).

4. Dan Millman, *Way of the Peaceful Warrior: A Book That Changes Lives* (CA, New World Library, 1980).

5. Lemberg, *Be Unreasonable*, 1.

6. *Vision Quest*. Dir. Harold Becker. Perfs. Matthew Modine, Linda Fiorentino. Warner Bros. Pictures, 1985.

7. Rick Warren, *The Purpose Driven Life* (Grand Rapids, MI, Zondervan, 2002).

8. Shunryu Suzuki, *Zen Mind, Beginner's Mind* (Boston, MA, Shambhala, 2011), 21.

Works Cited

Dyer, Dr. Wayne. 2004. *The Power of Intention*. India: Hay House.

Lemberg, Paul. 2007. *Be Unreasonable: The Unconventional Way to Extraordinary Business Results*. New York: McGraw-Hill Education.

Lipton, Bruce H. 2008. *The Biology of Belief: Unleashing the Power of Consciousness, Matter and Miracles*. India: Hay House.

Millman, Dan. 1980. *Way of the Peaceful Warrior: A Book That Changes Lives*. California: New World Library.

Modine, Matthew. *Vision Quest*. DVD. Directed by Harold Becker. Burbank: Warner Bros. Pictures, 1985.

Suzuki, Shunryu. 2011. *Zen Mind, Beginner's Mind*. Boston: Shambhala.

Warren, Rick. 2002. *The Purpose Driven Life*. Grand Rapids: Zondervan.